You're Not Broken-You're Unbalanced

Gain your life back by balancing hormones, restoring energy, improving sleep, and rebuilding metabolic health

Travis Woodley, MSN, RN, CRNP

Full Medical & Legal Disclaimer

This book—*You're Not Broken, You're Unbalanced*—is an educational resource. It is **not** medical advice and does **not** create a patient–provider relationship with the authors, editors, or publisher. Although many examples refer to midlife and menopause, the material addresses physiology across life stages and for all genders; how (or whether) any concept applies to you is an individual medical decision.

The supplement tables, sample protocols, and dosing ranges are **informational only** and may be incomplete, outdated, or inappropriate for your situation. Nutritional supplements, peptides, exosomes, bioidentical hormones (BHRT), lifestyle programs, and any other therapies discussed can interact with medications and medical conditions and may have risks, contraindications, and side effects.

Before starting, stopping, or changing **any** medication, supplement, peptide therapy, hormone therapy, exercise, or nutrition plan referenced in this book, consult a licensed healthcare professional who can evaluate your personal medical history, current prescriptions, allergies, and lab results; order appropriate baseline testing; and provide follow-up care. Never disregard professional medical advice or delay seeking it because of something you read here.

Statements about dietary supplements have **not** been evaluated by the U.S. Food and Drug Administration. Supplements are **not intended to diagnose, treat, cure, or prevent any disease**. Regulatory status for some therapies (e.g., peptides/exosomes) varies by jurisdiction; follow local laws and professional guidance.

The authors, contributors, and publisher disclaim all liability for any loss or damage resulting from the use of information in this book. Use of this content is at your own risk.

How Revitalize Aesthetics & Wellness Gave Us Our Marriage Back

When my wife, Donna, and I first met, life felt effortless. We dated with ease, married with joy, and started our years together with hope. Somewhere along the way, that ease slipped. It wasn't one big event; it was a series of small drifts—shorter tempers, lighter sleep, heavier bodies, quieter desire. We found ourselves arguing about things that didn't matter and avoiding the things that did. Eventually we were living mostly apart, and when we were together, it felt like we were waiting for the next explosion. We loved each other, but love was losing ground to exhaustion.

We were both carrying more weight than we wanted. We weren't exercising. We ate for comfort and convenience, and we told ourselves we were "just getting older." Deep down, I prayed for change—specifically for our marriage, and also for the energy and hope to rebuild it. A trusted friend told us about her best friend's experience with bioidentical hormone optimization and how it transformed not just her energy, but her relationship. Skeptical but desperate for a path forward, we booked a comprehensive evaluation with Travis Woodley, MSN, RN, CRNP, and his team at Revitalize Aesthetics & Wellness.

From the first appointment, we knew we were in the right place. Travis didn't offer quick fixes or generic advice. He listened. He explained how hormones are the body's master messengers—how sleep, mood, metabolism, and even patience and intimacy follow those signals—and how "normal" lab ranges don't always align with how people feel or function. For the first time, our symptoms were treated like meaningful data, not inconveniences to medicate away.

With Travis's guidance, we chose to begin bioidentical hormone therapy and, based on our lifestyle and preference, selected pellet delivery to support steady levels. We paired this with simple, practical choices we could live with: protein-forward eating, consistent bedtime, daily walking, and eventually, strength training together. Nothing changed overnight. But something quieter began—fewer blowups, more patience, lighter mornings. That was enough to keep going.

Over the next several weeks, the momentum grew. Energy rose. Brain fog lifted. Workouts felt possible, then enjoyable. We started cooking real food and eating with intention. Affection returned in small, tender ways, and intimacy followed—not just because desire woke up, but because we felt like teammates again. Donna, who never thought of herself as a morning person, met me at the gym before sunrise. I watched her strength and confidence return, one set at a time. My weight dropped steadily; my composition improved; I recognized myself again—not because the clock turned back, but because our biology finally started working with us instead of against us.

It wasn't effortless. We showed up on days we didn't feel like it. We made our follow-ups. We stayed coachable. We also prayed—often. And we are profoundly grateful: to Travis for his leadership and compassion, to the Revitalize Aesthetics & Wellness team for their care, and to a plan that honored both science and real life. We didn't just get lab numbers in a better range—we got our marriage back.

Why open this book with our story? Because what you're about to read is the roadmap we wish we'd had sooner. Travis lays out, with clarity and empathy, how to read your body's signals and what to do about them—how hormone optimization, sleep, nutrition, stress rhythm, muscle, peptides, and high-quality nutraceuticals fit together as one system. He explains why the answers many of us were given—"normal labs," "try to relax," "that's aging"—didn't match what our bodies were telling us.

If you're discouraged, skeptical, or simply tired, please hear this: there is real hope here. You don't have to become a biochemist. You need a clinician who listens, a plan that respects cause-and-effect, and a sequence that fits your life. Our results are our own, but the pattern is repeatable: align the signals, supply the materials, remove the friction, protect the rhythms, and show up long enough for momentum to take over.

Today, Donna and I plan our future with energy and affection. We cook differently. We sleep differently. We train together before work. We argue less and laugh more. We miss each other when we're apart. The fact that we can say all of that after where we were is a gift we won't take for granted.

Travis, thank you for writing this book and for the work you and your team do every day. Revitalize Aesthetics & Wellness didn't just improve our numbers—it restored our balance and reminded us who we are together. If you're holding this book and standing where we once stood, let this be your sign: keep reading, take the first step, and allow yourself to believe that your best years are not behind you.

With gratitude and hope,

Craig S.

on behalf of my wife, Donna

Note: Our story reflects our experience under the care of Travis Woodley, MSN, RN, CRNP, and the team at Revitalize Aesthetics & Wellness. Every patient is different. This foreword is not medical advice; consult your healthcare provider before making changes.

Medical & Ethical Disclosures

Medical Disclaimer

This book is for educational purposes only and is not a substitute for individualized medical advice, diagnosis, or treatment. Reading this book does not create a patient–provider relationship. Do not start, stop, or change medications, supplements, or procedures without consulting a qualified clinician who can review your health history, labs, and current therapies.

Supplement & Peptide Notices

Statements regarding nutraceuticals describe structure/function support (e.g., helps maintain, supports, promotes) and are not intended to diagnose, treat, cure, or prevent disease. Peptides and certain procedures may be used off-label under medical supervision; quality, identity, and dosing should be verified through reputable, lawful sources. Outcomes vary.

Procedural Acknowledgments

O-Shot® and P-Shot® are associated with Charles Runels, MD. These procedures are not FDA-cleared for specific indications; discuss risks, benefits, and alternatives with your clinician.

Table of Contents

Foreword By Dr. Derrick M. DeSilva, Jr., M.D

We are aware that the seven dwarves of menopause are Itchy, Bitchy, Sleepy, Sweaty, Bloated, Forgetful, and Psycho. Menopause, a significant life transition for women and is a profound change in life. This "life shift" not only affects women but also their families, friends, and loved ones who surround them.

The important thing for a woman heading towards menopause is to realize that knowledge is power. When menopause begins, instead of allowing mood swings and feelings of irritation to consume you, you should recognize it as a necessary physiological process and know that you are not alone. There is help available as you navigate this new phase of your life. This book will be your roadmap as you navigate this journey called menopause.

Some women feel less excitement towards sex and intimacy. It's normal for women to feel depressed, anxious, stressed, experience bladder problems, disturbed sleep, thinning hair, loss of memory, weight gain, and so much more. It's generally around this time that the children have reached an age where they are ready to move on with their independent lives, and dealing with the emotions of an empty-nest syndrome. Instead of solely battling an onslaught of emotions, physiological changes, mental breakdowns etc, it will be much easier if you AND your family members are made aware of the nature of this process. This book is not only for the woman who is managing the journey of menopause, but it is also for the husband and significant other who is involved in "that woman's" life. This phase of life is a journey that needs to be navigated with understanding, love, and support.

As a physician working in this field for many decades, this journey that women go through is likely one of the most difficult and most misunderstood physiological processes. Some women sail through the years of menopause, and others sit in front of me and immediately start to cry and cannot control their emotions. So what is the process? And how do you maneuver and navigate this process during this very difficult time in life? As you read through this book, the road map for you will become clear. You do have many options when it comes to safe and effective hormone replacement therapy. There are also many myths around hormone replacement therapy. The hormone replacement therapy that I am talking about and that will be discussed in this book is called bioidentical hormone replacement therapy or BHRT. When you look at the words bioidentical hormone replacement therapy, it should immediately become obvious to you that the hormones that are given or replaced are biologically identical to what your body produces. This therapy has been shown to be effective in managing the symptoms of menopause. But bioidentical hormone replacement therapy (BHRT) it's only a piece of the puzzle. Women must take responsibility for what they consume as their fuel for their bodies, along with movement and basic nutrient replenishment. As you read through the chapters the details of each one of these modalities will be explained in much more detail. But there's more to this story. When I speak with my patients about all of the pieces to the puzzle, I also introduce a spiritual component that I believe should be a part everyone's life. I'm not talking about going to church every day I am simply talking about being a good person and doing that daily good deed. The daily good deed is one of the most important and scientifically proven actions to help support the health of your immune system. Once again, there's more to the story, along with feeding your body, movement, and basic nutrient supplementation along with new therapies such as peptides and exosomes could also be part of this "healing" process.

As I previously mentioned, you have options as to how bioidentical hormones can be utilized by you. Some of the delivery mechanisms that will be discussed are creams, pellets, sublinguals, and injections. Most women use either creams, pellets, or sublinguals. Most women do not use injections to deliver hormones. Injections are utilized mostly by men to deliver testosterone due to the higher doses of testosterone that are required by men. Each one of these modalities has its benefits And can be customized to your lifestyle. The way you choose to receive your bioidentical hormones is a discussion that you need to have with your provider.

The one thing that I will stress is that you find an experienced provider that has been trained and understands how to properly use bioidentical hormones and also, more importantly, knows how to dose and manage any potential complications. If this therapy is dosed properly, the complications will be minimized. What I have seen over the past many decades is that there are many practitioners who do bioidentical hormone replacement therapy for the wrong reasons. They are poorly trained, and what I have seen in many hormone practices absolutely frightens me. Many clinics have popped up all over the country that prescribe bio-identical hormone replacement therapy, but the practitioner has little to no training. I have seen many women and men who have been dosed inappropriately and have been given therapies that were not necessary. The appropriate lab work and regular follow-ups with a real practitioner are, in my opinion, the key to successfully navigating this journey called menopause. Most of the clinics do not order the correct blood work, the appropriate radiologic tests, specifically a mammogram and a transvaginal ultrasound, prior to starting bioidentical hormone replacement therapy. Establishing the correct baselines for women is a very important piece of this therapy. I read an article in Scientific American that was published in 2025 on the role of testosterone therapy in men. The bottom line of that article was that most practitioners are doing hormone replacement therapy for the wrong reason. The wrong reason is mainly financial and not for the total care of the patient. This not only goes for men but also for women. The management of bioidentical hormone replacement therapy for men, in my opinion, is very simple. The management of bioidentical hormone replacement therapy in women is much more complicated. In a woman, we are managing 5 hormones. The hormones that we are managing in a woman are estrogen, progesterone, testosterone, thyroid, and cortisol. If these hormones are not managed synchronously, the outcomes are not going to be optimal. Once again, I will stress that you use this book as a road map through your journey called menopause. Do your homework and make sure that you ask the right questions, you have the right testing done before starting bioidentical hormone replacement therapy, and make sure that regular follow-ups are done with a well-trained, experienced practitioner. The bottom line is that you are ultimately responsible for your own health. Books like this will help you navigate this journey called menopause, and once you have a good road map for this journey, you will be able to reach that goal of optimal health. Enjoy this very well-written road map and remember that there's no need for you to be one of the seven dwarves of menopause.

May You Always be Blessed with Good Health.

In The Author's Words

I'm grateful to Derrick M. DeSilva, Jr., M.D. for lending his voice to this project. For decades he has cared for patients while bridging Eastern and Western medicine, teaching clinicians, and speaking in national forums—all with a single aim: give people the best of both worlds and help them feel well again.

This book was born from thousands of conversations with people who felt "off" and were told it was "just aging" or "just stress." I've sat with women navigating perimenopause and menopause, and with men whose strength, drive, and focus were quietly slipping. I've met couples who love each other but feel like roommates because energy and desire have been running on empty. And I've seen, again and again, that these patterns are not moral failings. They're signals—chemistry asking to be heard.

You're not broken. You're out of balance. When the body's messenger system drifts—estrogen, progesterone, testosterone, thyroid, DHEA, cortisol—everything downstream works harder. Sleep fractures. Mood and focus blur. Insulin gets noisy, weight creeps, hair and skin change, confidence fades. The way back isn't a single hack or a louder stimulant; it's a sequence: restore the signals, supply the materials, remove friction, protect your daily rhythms, and measure what actually matters in your life—sleep, energy, mood, cognition, body composition, and intimacy.

Sometimes bioidentical hormone replacement therapy (BHRT) is part of that plan—not to make you someone else, but to give your cells the same clear instructions they understood years ago, safely and in amounts that fit you. You'll also meet peptides—small, targeted signals your body already speaks—that can, when used judiciously and in partnership with a qualified clinician, help good habits stick and momentum return. But the biggest wins so often start with foundations: protein-forward, minimally processed nutrition; micronutrients that close repair gaps; muscle-building movement; a protect-your-sleep routine; and practical tools to calm an over-revved nervous system. Throughout these pages, we'll keep solutions evidence-aware, real-life-friendly, and free of shame or scare tactics.

This isn't a book of shortcuts. It's a blueprint for capacity. I'll ask you to get smarter labs and learn what they mean. I'll invite you to personalize instead of copy someone else's plan. And I'll be frank about trade-offs: BHRT should be individualized and monitored; peptides should be sourced responsibly and used within a larger plan; and supplements should be targeted and high-quality—because more is not better; better is better. Conventional medicine remains essential. This book isn't anti-medicine; it's pro-root cause, pro-prevention, and pro-partnership—combining the best of standard care with the best of restorative strategies so you function and feel like yourself again.

If you've felt dismissed, consider this your microphone. If you've felt overwhelmed, this is your simplifier—one chapter at a time, one lever at a time. Biology forgives quickly when you give it what it's been asking for. In weeks, sleep can deepen. In months, strength and focus return. Over a year, your labs—and your daily life—can tell a different story. Start where it matters most to you. Track lightly. Adjust with your clinician. Let small, consistent wins compound.

Read with a pen. Circle what sounds like your story. Bring good questions to a qualified provider. Most of all, begin. You're not broken—you're out of balance. Balance can be rebuilt.

Disclosure & Release: Derrick M. DeSilva, Jr., M.D. involvement with this work is limited to authoring the foreword. He did not author, edit, or review the remainder of the manuscript, the protocols, or any product mentions. His foreword reflects his professional perspective and is offered for general education only; it does not constitute medical advice, does not establish a patient–provider relationship, and should not be relied upon for diagnosis or treatment. To the fullest extent permitted by law, Derrick M. DeSilva, Jr., M.D. assumes no responsibility or liability for any use of information contained in this book. **Compensation disclosure:** Derrick M. DeSilva, Jr., M.D. received **no compensation** for authoring the foreword. He holds no ownership interest in, and receives no royalties, affiliate commissions, or product proceeds from, this book or from any product or service referenced herein.

With respect and optimism,

Travis Woodley, MSN, RN, CRNP
Author, *You're Not Broken—You're Out of Balance*

Introduction

If you're holding this book, there's a good chance you've already felt it—the quiet drift from the way you remember feeling to the way you feel now. Mornings take longer to start. Sleep shows up when it wants to. Workouts don't "pay you back" like they used to. Your mind can be crystal clear one moment and foggy the next. You're not lazy, weak, or undisciplined. You're not broken. You're out of balance.

That word—balance—isn't a slogan. It's physiology. Your body runs on messages: hormones that tell cells when to repair, when to grow, when to burn, when to rest. Your brain, gut, muscles, bones, blood vessels, and immune system all listen in. When the messages are strong and synchronized, everyday life feels surprisingly easy. When they fade or fall out of rhythm, everything asks for more effort. You push harder, but the returns get smaller. Most people are told to accept this as "getting older," and then they're handed a stack of prescriptions to manage symptoms one by one. That's not health; that's maintenance. This book offers something better: a map for getting the messages back.

You'll notice the tone here is plainspoken and practical. We're going to talk about bioidentical hormone replacement therapy (BHRT) in a way that demystifies it—what it is, how it differs from synthetics, who it's right for, and how it's personalized. We'll explore peptide therapy as a set of precision tools for healing and performance—short, targeted signals that help your body do what it's already designed to do. We'll look hard at nutrition—not as calorie math but as information—because food either calms your biology or keeps it on high alert. We'll repair the gut, because your microbiome and intestinal lining don't just affect digestion; they help set your mood, your immune tone, your estrogen metabolism, your cravings, and your inflammation baseline. We'll restore sleep and circadian rhythm so your brain and tissues can actually integrate the gains you work for during the day. We'll build muscle on purpose, because muscle is not vanity—it's glucose control, joint protection, mitochondrial density, and a live-longer organ. We'll bring in medical-grade nutraceuticals where they matter, not as a multivitamin blanket, but as targeted support for pathways that lab work and symptoms tell us need help.

Underneath all of that is a simple promise: the way you feel is not random. There are reasons. And when you address the reasons in the right order, your biology becomes easier to live in.

You will also hear a clear critique of the model many of us were raised in. The pharmaceutical industry saves lives every day in emergencies; that's not in dispute. But a system built to code and bill for diagnoses will always be better at managing late-stage problems than preventing them. The same processed food economy that fills our shelves also fills our clinics—because ultra processed grains, industrial seed oils, and sugar keep inflammation high, insulin jumpy, and appetite dysregulated. That combination is great for repeat business and terrible for health span. You deserve the whole story and the tools to step outside of that loop.

Think of this book as a conversation with a clinician who has stood at both bedsides: the hospital bed and the kitchen table. We'll translate lab values into lived experience. "Normal" ranges will be unpacked so you understand the gap between average and optimal. You'll learn why women and men both need testosterone (at different levels), why estrogen is protective far beyond hot flashes, why progesterone is a sleep and calm hormone as much as a uterine one, and why thyroid conversion (T4 → T3) can make or break your metabolism and mood. We'll talk about DHEA as resilience. We'll explain why estradiol and testosterone delivered in steady ways can transform daily life—and why the right route, dose, and follow-up matter more than hype.

You'll meet peptides with specific jobs: compounds that nudge growth hormone pulses for deeper sleep and better recovery; signals that help tendons, ligaments, and gut lining actually heal; mitochondrial helpers that make movement feel lighter and energy steadier; brain-supporting blends that sharpen focus and motivation during transitions. You'll see how they integrate with BHRT rather than replace it—because replacing missing messages and amplifying repair are different, complementary jobs.

Nutrition will be reframed as signal design. Protein isn't just "macros"; it's the raw material for muscle, enzymes, neurotransmitters, and immune components. Colorful plants aren't just "fiber"; they carry polyphenols that calm oxidative stress and support detox pathways, including the ones that decide how you metabolize estrogen. Healthy fats aren't villains; they're the backbone for steroid hormones and the building blocks of cell membranes where all those hormone receptors live. We'll make food practical—plates you can build, not rules you can break.

Gut health gets its own spotlight because it's the switchboard between your outside world and your inside one. When the lining is tight and the microbial community is balanced, nutrients land where they should, the immune system stays appropriately calm, and the "estrobolome" (gut bacteria involved in estrogen metabolism) behaves. When that system leaks or overgrows, you don't just get bloating—you get inflammation that blunts hormone signaling, cravings that aren't "willpower" problems, skin that flares, and moods that swing. We'll walk through staged resets that remove irritants, bind and escort offenders, and rebuild the mucosal barrier. You'll understand why targeted immunoglobulins, minerals, B-vitamins in methylated forms, omega-3s, magnesium, and vitamins A/D/K can be difference-makers—not because they're trendy, but because they support the exact chemistry you're trying to restore.

Sleep is the quiet superpower threading through every chapter. Deep, consolidated sleep is where your brain clears waste, memory consolidates, muscles repair, insulin sensitivity resets, and hormone timing re-synchronizes. We'll treat it like a medical intervention: light timing, temperature, caffeine cutoffs, wind-down design, and (when needed) short, supervised peptide support while the habits take hold. If you've been told to "just relax," you'll get something better: a stepwise plan that gives your nervous system permission to downshift again.

Strength training isn't optional if you care about aging well. You'll learn why two to three weekly sessions—push, pull, hinge, squat, carry—plus daily walking outperform any pill for sarcopenia, glucose control, and mood. We'll cover how optimized hormones make training feel rewarding again, how connective-tissue support reduces injury fear, and how mitochondria multiply in response to the right dose of effort.

A word on fear: you may have heard unsettling things about hormone therapy—rumors that don't match modern, individualized use of bioidentical hormones. We'll clarify what's signal and what's noise, how route and dose shape risk/benefit, what to monitor, and how to adjust. You'll never be asked to "believe"; you'll be invited to understand and then decide.

What about cost? There's an honest answer here, too. There is a cost to doing nothing—we just pay it in slow motion. Poor sleep taxes your mood, memory, and relationships. Muscle loss taxes your joints and independence. Ignoring insulin resistance taxes your brain, your arteries, and your confidence. Shifting resources toward food that nourishes, plans that fit, and care that treats causes is not indulgence; it's a reallocation with compounding returns.

How to use this book: start where your biggest friction lives. If sleep is broken, begin there and protect it ruthlessly. If energy crashes define your days, address insulin and mitochondrial capacity first. If pain keeps you from moving, fix the tissues and the inflammatory noise so you can train. If mood and motivation feel dulled, bring hormones back to functional ranges and give your brain the nutrients and rhythms it needs to light up. Use the symptom-to-strategy tables and case stories as orientation, not as rigid recipes. Your plan should look like you: your goals, your labs, your schedule, your budget, your season of life.

A note on personalization and safety: nothing here replaces a thoughtful evaluation by a qualified clinician who understands optimization, not just crisis care. BHRT requires individualized dosing and follow-up. Peptides should be sourced through reputable medical channels. Supplements should be professional-grade and third-party tested. This book will help you ask better questions, recognize quality, and partner effectively with your care team.

Finally, expect momentum. Biology loves clarity. When you clean up signals and sequence the work—restore hormones, repair the gut, rebuild muscle, re-train sleep, reduce inflammatory load—your body responds faster than you think it can. The first wins are often subtle: fewer nighttime wake-ups, steadier mornings, a workout that feels "right" again, a calmer relationship with food, a laugh that comes more easily. Then the labs catch up: fasting insulin and CRP drift down, thyroid conversion improves, lipids shift in the direction of health, sex hormones sit where you actually feel like yourself. That's not a miracle. That's physiology—finally getting the inputs it's been asking for.

If you've felt dismissed, talked over, or handed medications without a map, I wrote this for you. If you're a clinician who suspects there's a more humane way to practice than chase symptoms, I wrote it for you, too. We can do better than managed decline. We can build health on purpose.

Turn the page. Let's get your balance back.

Chapter 1

The New Era of Aging Well: Why Decline Is a Choice, Not a Destiny

She gripped the bathroom counter and studied the woman in the mirror. The face was familiar but quieter somehow—eyes a little duller, jaw set a little tighter, skin not quite keeping up with how she felt inside. Emily was forty-nine and good at pretending she was fine. She led projects at work, volunteered at her kids' school, kept track of birthdays and dentist appointments and oil changes. But lately she could feel her edges fraying. Nights were light and broken—hot flashes that came like waves, a mind that wouldn't stop listing the next day's tasks—so mornings started already behind. Coffee bought her a few hours, then the afternoon fog rolled in and the world turned to static. Her joints pinched when she stood up. Her jeans fit differently. Sex had shifted from natural to negotiable. And the most surprising part wasn't the changes themselves; it was that the people she asked for help acted like this was the deal she had signed up for. "It's just getting older," her doctor said. "Happens to everyone."

What Emily felt is not rare; it is the most common story of midlife. We absorb a cultural script that says decline is "natural," and the polite, reasonable thing to do is accept it. We are offered prescriptions for sleep, mood, blood pressure, and cholesterol—sometimes for symptoms caused by other prescriptions—and we are told to be grateful for maintenance. Meanwhile supermarket aisles glow with processed convenience, and we try to ignore the way those foods leave us hungrier and more tired than before. When you step back, it's hard to miss the pattern: a system that waits for you to break, then sells you a brace.

Here is a better truth: aging is inevitable; decline is optional. Your body is not a machine with an expiration date; it is a living system designed to repair, remodel, and adapt. The friction most of us call "aging" is, in large part, the compounded effect of misaligned inputs—hormones drifting out of the ranges where we feel best, mitochondria under-fueled and over-stressed, inflammation quietly smoldering, sleep shortened and fragmented, food that signals chaos instead of stability. Realignment is not wishful thinking. It's a process grounded in physiology and reinforced by thousands of lived results.

If you strip away the noise, there are two kinds of age. Chronological age is the count of birthdays. Biological age is how old you truly function. You have met the forty-five-year-old who moves like sixty and the sixty-eight-year-old who moves like forty. The difference is not luck. It's the sum of what they ask of their bodies and what they give their bodies in return—hormonal balance, nutrient density, movement, stress rhythm, sleep architecture. The promise of this book is simple: when you work with those levers, you move your biological age in the direction you want to live.

Another distinction matters just as much: lifespan versus healthspan. Lifespan counts years. Healthspan counts the years you wake up clear, move easily, think sharply, and feel at home in your body. Many people spend their final fifteen to twenty years managing diseases they never wanted and taking medications to counter the effects of other medications. That story can be edited. If you extend the part of life that is healthy and capable, you reclaim experiences that matter most—travel without dragging, dancing at your child's wedding, picking up grandkids without bracing, work that still feels like purpose, intimacy that still feels alive.

Let's return to Emily. When she finally decided that "just aging" wasn't an answer, she asked for a different kind of evaluation. Comprehensive labs replaced quick glances. Instead of being told she was "in the normal range," she learned the difference between normal and optimal. Her estrogen and progesterone had fallen well below the zone where sleep is stable and mood is elastic. Her free testosterone—yes, women make and need it—was almost undetectable, which explained the shrinking muscle tone and flat libido. Her thyroid looked "okay" by conventional thresholds, but conversion to its active form lagged. Inflammation markers were high from years of rushed meals and interrupted rest. What she needed was not a larger pill organizer. She needed her body's messaging system restored, her cells' energy engines refueled, and her daily inputs simplified to support repair instead of sabotage.

Bioidentical hormone replacement therapy (BHRT) was the first lever. "Bioidentical" simply means the molecules match what the body recognizes. Hormones are your internal emails—tiny messengers that tell cells what to do and when to do it. When those messages get quiet, everything gets confused: you store fat instead of burning it, build less muscle from the same workout, sleep lightly, worry more, and recover slowly. Restoring hormones to youthful, functional ranges does not make you someone you're not; it allows you to be yourself again, with the volume turned back up to where your body runs clean.

The second lever was targeted repair signals—peptides. Peptides are short chains of amino acids the body uses like post-it notes for specific jobs. Some peptides remind your tissues to heal; some remind your brain to focus; some nudge your metabolism toward fat-burning; others calm inflammation. Because they work with existing pathways rather than bulldozing them, they tend to play nicely with the body, amplifying what you want without creating new problems to solve. BPC-157 supports gut lining integrity and tendon and ligament recovery, so meals land more gently and joints feel more trusting. TB500 helps tissues remodel after years of micro-injury. AOD9604 encourages fat cells to let go of stored energy without spiking growth hormone. PT-141, acting centrally, can reawaken desire in both men and women without tinkering with sex hormone levels. GHK-Cu tells skin and hair follicles that renewal is on the agenda. NAD+ and BDNF blends support cellular energy and neuroplasticity, turning down the fog.

Third came the raw materials: nutraceuticals that are more than generic multivitamins. Think of ADK10—a combination of vitamins A, D3, and K2—as permission slips for bone and cardiovascular tissue to use minerals wisely, and for hormone receptors to listen better. Omega-3s (in balanced EPA/DHA forms like Super Omega 3D) help quiet the fires of inflammation and support the brain that navigates your whole day. Magnesium (as in Mag Complete) is the mineral of "calm" chemistry, involved in hundreds of reactions that govern muscle relaxation, sleep depth, and insulin sensitivity. Gut-support formulas like GI Complete help knit the intestinal lining so the nutrients you eat actually become the tissues you need. When overgrowths like candida or parasites are part of the fatigue-and-bloating puzzle, targeted botanicals and nutrients—protocols akin to CandiKill and ParaKill—can reset the terrain. Where thyroid drag is part of the picture, comprehensive formulas resembling Thyroid Complete supply the cofactors that allow the gland's signals to be understood. When stress chemistry has been redlined for too long, adaptogenic blends comparable to AdrenaMax or Adrenal Restore help the body remember how to downshift without crashing. And for foundational coverage, men's and women's comprehensive blends can fill the micronutrient gaps our modern food leaves.

Fourth came the rhythms: sleep that arrives and stays, movement that builds instead of breaks, meals that stabilize instead of spike. Emily learned that building and protecting muscle is not vanity; it's health insurance. Muscle is an organ of longevity—one that disposes of glucose, stabilizes joints, sends anti-inflammatory signals (myokines), and stores amino acids for emergencies. Two to three sessions a week of smart strength training became non-negotiable, with daily walking as the simplest form of recovery and metabolic support. She learned that blue light at midnight is not a harmless habit; it's a message to stay alert when her body wants to repair. She learned that protein at breakfast stabilizes the whole day, that cruciferous vegetables help the body metabolize estrogens cleanly, that healthy fats are not villains but building blocks for hormones and cell membranes, and that removing ultra-processed grains and seed oils is not a punishment but a relief.

Within eight weeks the changes felt impossible to ignore. Night sweats evaporated. Sleep consolidated into deep, restoring cycles. Mornings stopped feeling like a hangover without the night before. Her husband noticed she laughed more easily. Her kids noticed she said yes to walks after dinner. The scale began to shift not because she ate less of everything, but because she ate more of the right things—food that told her body it was safe to burn what it had been storing. At six months, her lab work matched what she felt: hormones in optimal ranges, inflammation quieter, thyroid signals more responsive, lipids improved, fasting glucose steady. She didn't become a different person. She became herself again.

Did You Know? The lab range called "normal" only describes the average of everyone who gets tested. In midlife, many people in those datasets already feel poorly. "Optimal" is the range where people report feeling and functioning best. The difference between those two words can be the difference between coping and thriving.

If you have been told your hormones are "fine," consider what that actually means. Often it means you sit somewhere inside a very wide net. A forty-nine-year-old woman with estrogen just above the threshold for "low" and progesterone barely detectable might be told she is "within normal limits," even as she wakes three times a night, snaps at the people she loves, and watches motivation slide. A fifty-two-year-old man with testosterone at 310 ng/dL might hear "normal" while he feels his confidence and muscle erode. Normal is a population curve. Optimal is a life you want to live.

Decline loves confusion. It thrives when you're told different stories by different experts and end up frozen between them. One authority says fat is the enemy; another says carbs are the enemy; another says "eat everything in moderation" while your body begs for a better plan. One suggests a sleeping pill to force sleep; another prescribes a stimulant to force wakefulness. But biology isn't a set of isolated switches. It's a network. When estrogen falls, sleep and mood suffer. When sleep suffers, insulin sensitivity drops. When insulin sensitivity drops, the body holds onto fat and releases more inflammatory signals. When inflammation rises, hormone receptors become less responsive. The good news is that the network works in your favor too. Restore hormones, and sleep deepens. Sleep deepens, and blood sugar steadies. Blood sugar steadies, and inflammation cools. Inflammation cools, and receptors listen better. Momentum compounds either way. Choose your slope.

Did You Know? Your muscles talk to your brain. During and after resistance training, muscles release myokines—signals that reduce inflammation, support neuroplasticity, and improve insulin sensitivity. In practice, that means the right kind of training doesn't just sculpt your body; it sharpens your mind and steadies your mood.

Maybe you're wondering where medications fit. There is a time and place for pharmaceuticals; they can be lifesaving and bridge difficult seasons. But the dominant model many of us were raised in is reactive: wait for a diagnosis code, then match a drug. It manages crisis better than it creates health. Pills for blood pressure and blood sugar and mood are often necessary in emergencies, but they do not rebuild the physiology that got frayed. The approach outlined in this book goes under the symptom and asks "why." Why did sleep come apart? Why did the weight gather around the middle? Why did the appetite tilt toward sweets at night? Why did the focus dull at 3 p.m.? The answers usually live in hormones, mitochondria, inflammation, micronutrients, and rhythm—the places you can influence every day.

Consider Marcus, sixty-two, who used to be the hardest worker on any job site. He wasn't ill, exactly, but he wasn't himself. By late afternoon his hands felt thick; his knees asked him to reconsider stairs; his memory for names—the one thing he'd always prided himself on—faded at the edges. His labs told a familiar story: testosterone at "low-normal," estradiol too low to protect joints, DHEA depleted, vitamin D in the basement, fasting insulin creeping up, CRP elevated. He began BHRT with careful attention to both testosterone and estradiol balance (men need some estrogen for joints, vessels, and brain), brought strength training back as a prescription instead of a hobby, and supported recovery with peptides—CJC-1295 paired with Ipamorelin to revive growth hormone pulses, BPC-157 for an old shoulder that had quietly limited his reach, MOTS-C with AICAR to remind his mitochondria what efficient felt like. He learned to eat protein first and often, to respect sleep like a meeting with his future self, and to take magnesium at night like a key that fits a lock. Nine months later he wasn't trying to be thirty again; he was building a strong sixty-two. His crew noticed he moved faster. His wife noticed he laughed more. He noticed he didn't think about the stairs anymore.

Did You Know? Estrogen is not just a "female" hormone and testosterone is not just a "male" hormone. Both sexes make and need both—at different levels—for brain protection, bone density, vascular health, sexual function, and mood.

At this point, you might already be matching your symptoms to your story. Perhaps your sleep feels shallow and you wake at 2:37 a.m. for no reason. Perhaps your appetite feels loud at night and quiet in the morning. Perhaps you find yourself avoiding intimacy not because you don't care but because you don't feel like you. Perhaps exercise leaves you more depleted than charged. If any of that sounds familiar, you're not broken. You're under-signaled and under-supplied.

What does "the new era of aging well" look like in practice? It looks like ordering comprehensive labs before life falls apart and using those results to guide action. It looks like treating nutrition as communication—protein to signal repair, colorful plants to signal detoxification and antioxidant defense, healthy fats to fortify cell membranes and produce hormones. It looks like reclaiming your evenings by dimming screens, cooling your bedroom, and letting your brain relearn darkness. It looks like strength training as a standing appointment with your long-term independence and walking as your daily moving meditation. It looks like using BHRT to restore messages, peptides to target repairs, and nutraceuticals to provide building blocks. It looks like noticing that your patience comes back before your waistline does—and that both follow.

People often ask, "Is this safe?" The better question is, "Is it safer than doing nothing?" We've normalized risk in one direction—risk of chronic disease, risk of fracture, risk of cognitive decline—while fixating on the risks of interventions that prevent them. BHRT, when individualized and monitored, is not a reckless experiment; it is a careful restoration of physiology. Peptides, when sourced responsibly and used judiciously, can amplify healing without the blunt force side effects many drugs carry. Nutraceuticals, when chosen for quality and purpose, are not random bottles but structural materials. Risk is real in both directions, which is why your plan should be personal, data-informed, and adjusted over time.

Did You Know? Sleep is the most affordable, widely available performance enhancer in the world. Deep sleep lengthens your healthspan by improving insulin sensitivity, consolidating memory, repairing muscle, clearing brain waste (via the glymphatic system), and resynchronizing your hormonal orchestra for the next day.

Emily's story didn't end with a single protocol; it unfolded as a series of choices that got easier because they worked. She started keeping promises to her future self: turning off screens by 9:30, walking after dinner, lifting on Mondays and Thursdays, eating a protein-forward breakfast, taking her magnesium with gratitude, honoring her labs with action rather than fear. Each piece reinforced the others. Her bedroom felt like a cave. Her refrigerator looked like a farm. Her calendar looked like a partnership between strength and recovery. This is what momentum feels like when it's pointed in your favor.

If you feel a flicker of optimism reading this, hold onto it. The point of this chapter is not to sell you a miracle; it's to hand you a map. The next chapters will turn that map into a route. We'll begin with the system that decides how everything else goes—the messenger network that tells your cells what to do, when to grow, when to repair, and when to rest. When hormones are tuned, life hums. When they drift, even the best intentions feel uphill. Understanding them is the hinge on which the door of healthspan swings.

Turn the page. The new era of aging well begins with the connection most of us were never taught to see: The Hormone Connection.

The reason this works—this shift from coping to building—is that you are correcting signals at their source. When hormones drift low, when inflammation stays high, when sleep stops behaving like sleep, the brain and body do not have the instructions they need to perform. Restoring those instructions is not cosmetic; it is foundational. Imagine running a company with broken email servers and missing project files. You can hold more meetings and work longer hours, but you won't solve the problem until the systems are fixed and the messages can get through.

In real life, that means step one is seeing clearly. The old habit is to wait until a crisis forces change. The new habit is to look under the hood before smoke appears. Comprehensive labs are lenses, not labels. They tell you how your thyroid is converting signals, how your sex hormones are balancing, how your cortisol rises and falls across the day, whether inflammation is whispering or shouting, and whether insulin is quietly keeping the peace or driving blood sugar swings. When you catch these patterns early, you can act before a crisis. When you've drifted for years, you can still act, but the arc back to balance is longer—so start now.

Did You Know? Skeletal muscle is the largest glucose sink in the body. More muscle means better blood sugar control, steadier energy, lower inflammation, and an easier time maintaining a healthy weight—independent of the scale. That's why strength training plus hormone optimization is a longevity force multiplier.

Let's give shape to the framework you will see throughout this book. Think of it as the Core Four—four pillars that work together so you can feel younger from the inside out. The first pillar is hormonal optimization. Hormones are the timekeepers of your physiology. In women, estrogen protects the brain, supports bone density, improves insulin sensitivity, and keeps tissues elastic; progesterone steadies mood, deepens sleep, and helps you feel safe in your own skin; testosterone builds and preserves muscle, supports confidence and drive, and protects against bone and metabolic decline. In men, testosterone maintains muscle and vigor, estradiol (at male levels) protects joints and vessels, progesterone tempers the nervous system, and thyroid sets the pace for all of it.

When those hormones return to functional ranges—yours, not your neighbor's—the lights come on. The second pillar is peptide precision. Peptides work like whispered reminders to systems that have fallen quiet. BPC-157 encourages tissues to seal and mend—gut lining, tendons, ligaments, muscle. TB500 reduces friction in inflamed or overused areas so you can train and live without the "aftershock." CJC-1295 + Ipamorelin nudges your own growth hormone rhythm back toward youthful, which is why recovery, lean mass, and fat metabolism improve when you pair it with strength training and sleep. MOTS-C with AICAR cues mitochondria to use fuel more efficiently so energy lasts longer without the jitters. PT-141 can reignite central arousal pathways without changing your sex hormone doses. GHK-Cu tells skin and hair follicles to repair and renew.

The third pillar is nutritional repatterning. Food is not only fuel; it is information. Highly processed carbohydrates and seed oils broadcast mayhem to your cells: spike insulin, store fat, inflame tissues, crave more. Protein-forward, colorful, minimally processed meals send an opposite message: build, repair, stabilize. Aim for protein at each meal to support muscle and hormones; add cruciferous vegetables to help your body process estrogen cleanly; choose fats that protect membranes—olive oil, avocado, nuts, seeds, pastured egg yolks, fatty fish—and limit the industrial oils that make membranes fragile and inflamed.

Did You Know? Ultra-processed foods now make up the majority of calories in many modern diets. They're engineered to be hyper-palatable and easy to overeat while providing little satiety or micronutrition. Your biology reads them as stress, not nourishment.

The fourth pillar is lifestyle synchronization—the daily rhythms that either magnify your efforts or muffle them. Sleep is where the deepest restoration happens: memory consolidates, hormones rebalance, immune cells patrol and repair. Treat bedtime like an appointment with tomorrow's clarity. Dim lights after dusk, cool your room, anchor your wake time. Movement should be both strategic and kind: two to three days of resistance training to protect muscle and bone; frequent walking to clear the mental cobwebs and steady blood sugar; mobility work to keep joints honest; a few joyful, breath-raising moments each day to remind your nervous system that you are alive and capable.

Now, let's anchor this in real lives. Ana, fifty-one, had been a night-shift nurse for years. She loved helping people, but the schedule took its toll: inverted sleep, sugar-heavy snacks to stay awake, no time to lift anything heavier than a chart. By the time she sought help, she was holding onto twenty extra pounds, waking with stiff hands, and forgetting details she never used to miss. Her labs showed the classic night-shift pattern: flattened cortisol rhythm, low estrogen and progesterone, low-normal thyroid hormones, and inflammatory markers that hummed like background noise. Restoring hormones, re-training her sleep window, adding a peptide cycle to support recovery, and prioritizing protein changed the texture of her days. Three months later, she wasn't perfect; she was moving forward—sleeping deeper on her nights off, lifting twice a week, and thinking clearly at 5 a.m.

Another story: DeShawn, fifty-eight, a contractor who prided himself on outworking men half his age. He noticed a quiet slide—grip weaker, belly thicker, energy shorter. He wasn't sick, but he wasn't himself. "Normal" labs said to wait and see. A deeper look said otherwise—testosterone and DHEA drifting low, estradiol too low for joint comfort, vitamin D bottoming out, fasting insulin creeping up, CRP elevated. He started with BHRT under a careful, individualized plan. CJC-1295 + Ipamorelin brought back restorative sleep and training response. Omega-3s, ADK10, and magnesium made recovery feel possible again. Twelve months later he didn't need an afternoon nap to be kind; he needed a walk because he had energy to spare.

Did You Know? Testosterone matters for women, too. In the right range, it supports mood, motivation, sexual desire, bone health, and the ability to build and preserve lean mass. "Low-normal" often isn't where women feel or function best.

If you are reading this and making a quiet list in your head—sleep that breaks, appetite that misbehaves, a mind that tires too soon—that is the point. Your body speaks in patterns more than in single symptoms. When multiple dials drift at once—hormones, sleep, inflammation, insulin—you don't need fifty fixes; you need the right sequence. Start by making noise where biology listens best: restore the messenger signals; provide the materials; remove the friction; protect the rhythms. The details vary by person, but the order often looks like this: sleep, hormones, protein and strength, gut repair, then fine-tuning with peptides and targeted supplementation.

Let's answer two questions that always arise. First: "Isn't this all complicated?" It looks that way from a distance. Up close, it's surprisingly orderly. You address one pillar at a time, in an order that makes sense for your body. Sometimes sleep is first, because without it nothing else sticks. Sometimes hormones are first, because without them you don't recover from training and don't want to cook nourishing meals. Sometimes gut repair is first, because without absorption your nutrients never arrive. Either way, momentum builds as the pieces reinforce each other.

Second: "Isn't this expensive?" There is a cost to doing nothing, and we rarely tally it. The slow tax of poor sleep is paid in mistakes and mood. The tax of muscle loss is paid in joint pain and lost independence. The tax of ignoring insulin resistance is paid in energy crashes, cravings, and future disease. None of this is a scare tactic; it's a reminder that you are already investing—either in decline by default or in vitality by design. Start where you can. Build from there. Many of the most potent changes cost little or nothing: morning light, walking after meals, lifting your own bodyweight, protein-forward meals cooked at home, earlier bedtimes, less alcohol on weeknights.

Did You Know? Morning light on your eyes (not through glass) anchors your circadian rhythm, making nighttime sleep deeper and hormone timing more precise. Ten minutes on a clear day—or thirty on a cloudy one—can change how your whole day feels.

If you are the kind of person who needs a first step, here are gentle ones that work across ages and seasons. Choose a protein-forward breakfast and walk for ten minutes afterward. Set a bedtime alarm that protects eight hours and keep screens out of the bedroom. Lift weights twice a week—nothing heroic, just consistent—and carry something heavy once a week (groceries count). Add magnesium in the evening and an omega-3 with your first meal. Ask for labs that look at function, not just survival—sex hormones (with free fractions), thyroid panel (including free T3), fasting insulin and glucose, lipids, CRP, vitamin D—and read them through the lens of how you actually feel.

This is how a new era begins—not with a single makeover, but with alignment. You are not late. Your biology responds quickly to respect. Within weeks, your sleep can deepen. Within months, your composition can shift. Within a year, your labs can look like they belong to a younger you. And the benefits stack—better sleep makes better food choices easier; better hormones make training feel rewarding; better gut health makes nutrients land where they're needed; better stress rhythm makes relationships easier.

Before we turn the page, return to Emily one last time. A year after she started, she doesn't check her phone to see how much she slept; she knows by how mornings feel. Work still asks a lot, but she has more to give without borrowing from tomorrow. She and her husband have Saturday morning coffee dates again—something that went missing when she felt like a dimmer switch turned down too low. She still has days, because everyone does, but the baseline—her sense of herself—is back. That is what this work provides.

You are capable of this. You are not fragile or behind. You are a system that responds to better inputs with better outputs. You don't have to memorize every mechanism to begin; you just have to understand the sequence and respect what your body is asking for. In the next chapter we will open the door that changes how the rest of the house looks and feels—the hormonal network that sets the tempo for your metabolism, your mood, your memory, your muscle, and your motivation. It's the connection most of us were never taught to see clearly.

Turn the page. Chapter 2 is where the map gets names and numbers: The Hormone Connection.

Chapter 2

The Hormone Connection

Your body runs on messages. A whisper from the brain to the ovaries, a signal from the adrenals to the immune system, a nudge from the thyroid to every cell that says, "Make energy." These messages are your hormones, and they set the tempo for how you think, feel, move, sleep, and heal. When the messages are strong and well-timed, life feels like it has traction. When they get faint or chaotic, you feel like you're pressing the gas in a car that won't shift out of second gear.

Most of us were never taught to see health this way. We were taught that symptoms are isolated events: hot flashes are separate from insomnia; brain fog has nothing to do with joint aches; low mood is a different story than belly fat. In reality, these are clusters that often trace back to the same control system: your hormones. This chapter is your map to that system—what each hormone does, what happens when it drifts, how to recognize the early flags, and how a thoughtful plan can bring the messengers back online.

We'll keep this simple and human. You don't need a medical degree to understand the signal-and-response logic that runs your body. You just need to know which dials matter, what "optimal" looks like in real life, and how to move in the right order: test, interpret, intervene, and re-assess.

The big six messengers for vitality are estrogen, progesterone, testosterone, DHEA, thyroid hormones (T4 and T3), and cortisol. They talk to one another constantly. Change one, and the others shift to compensate. That's why a single symptom rarely has a single cause. Think of them as instruments in an orchestra; when one goes flat, the entire performance sounds off.

Estrogen is the architect of fluidity and protection. In women, it supports brain wiring and memory, keeps tissues elastic, stabilizes blood sugar, protects bone, and fine-tunes vascular function. Men make estrogen too—from testosterone—and need it in a narrow range for joint comfort, libido, and cardiovascular health. When estrogen drops in women, hot flashes, night sweats, vaginal dryness, joint aches, and brain fog are common. Mood can feel brittle, and sleep becomes a light, broken thing. When estrogen is too low in men, joints can ache and libido can fade even if testosterone looks passable. When it runs too high relative to other hormones, water retention and breast tenderness can show up. The point isn't to chase a single number; it's to restore harmony.

Progesterone is the body's exhale. It builds calm, deepens sleep, and buffers the brain against stress. In the luteal phase of a woman's cycle and throughout the night, adequate progesterone is one of the reasons you fall asleep and stay there. When progesterone dips, anxiety climbs, patience thins, and sleep fragments—especially around 2–3 a.m. Restoring physiological levels often quiets that nocturnal wake-and-worry pattern, and paired with estrogen, it helps the nervous system feel safe again.

Testosterone is not just about muscle or sex; it's about drive. In women and men, it signals "build and repair"—supporting strength, resilience, motivation, cognition, and insulin sensitivity. When testosterone declines, effort feels heavier. Workouts produce more soreness than results. Belly fat collects even when calories haven't changed. Libido fades not only from mechanics but from low desire. In women, optimal (not male-level) testosterone supports mood, midsection leanness, and sexual satisfaction. In men, restoring physiological ranges brings back morning energy, decisiveness, and the willingness to train.

DHEA is a resilience hormone made by the adrenals. Think of it as a buffer for stress and a quiet supporter of immunity, libido, and mood. Low DHEA commonly rides alongside chronic stress, sleep loss, and heavy caffeine use. Bringing it back into range often smooths the rough edges of daily stress and complements testosterone and estrogen.

The thyroid is the thermostat of metabolism. The thyroid gland produces mostly T4, which must convert into T3—the active form—to light up energy production in your cells. When that conversion lags, you can see a normal TSH with a lowish free T3 and still feel textbook hypothyroid: cold hands and feet, dry skin, constipation, hair thinning, depression, and weight that clings. Supporting thyroid conversion—by correcting nutrient gaps, easing inflammation, improving sleep, and managing stress—often unlocks stubborn symptoms.

Cortisol is the rhythm keeper. You want it high in the morning to wake you and steadily lower toward evening so you can sleep. Chronically high cortisol feels like being wired and tired at once: anxious, snack-seeking, with belly fat that resists everything. Chronically low cortisol feels like a flat battery: slow mornings, salt cravings, and a short fuse. Because cortisol interacts with thyroid, sex hormones, and insulin, stabilizing its daily curve is one of the fastest ways to feel human again.

Now, how do these hormones drift out of range? Two main ways: time and friction. Time brings predictable changes—perimenopause and menopause in women; the slower slide of andropause in men. Friction is the modern world: ultra-processed food, sleep deprivation, stress without recovery, environmental chemicals, and too little muscle. The combination nudges the orchestra out of tune years earlier than it should.

The earliest signs are often brushed off: waking at 2:30 a.m. and staring at the ceiling, feeling tired but wired at night, needing caffeine to feel baseline, noticing workouts leave you more depleted than charged, losing your spontaneous desire for intimacy, experiencing unpredictable cycles, or losing your once-easy tolerance for stress. These are prompts, not punishments. Your body is flagging that the messenger system needs attention.

Because symptoms overlap and hormones interlock, testing is not optional—it's essential. "Treating the symptom" without reading the signals can make you feel worse. A smart baseline includes a sex hormone panel (total and free testosterone, estradiol using a sensitive assay, progesterone, DHEA-S, SHBG), a full thyroid panel (TSH, free T4, free T3, reverse T3, and thyroid antibodies when appropriate), adrenal rhythm testing (waking and diurnal cortisol pattern), metabolic markers (fasting insulin, fasting glucose, A1c), inflammation markers (hs-CRP), nutrient status (vitamin D, B12, folate, ferritin, magnesium), and safety screens tailored to the individual (PSA for men; appropriate breast and pelvic imaging for women based on age and history). You're not collecting trivia—you're drawing a map.

Once you can read that map, interventions make sense. Bioidentical hormone replacement therapy (BHRT) restores messaging with molecules your body recognizes. Delivery options—creams, injections, troches, and pellets—each have pros and cons, but the principle is the same: replace what's low to re-establish function. Contrary to widespread fear, personalized, monitored BHRT can be both safe and profoundly helpful when it brings hormones into physiologic ranges. The key is individualization and follow-up, not one-size-fits-all dosing.

Peptides are the second language of repair. CJC-1295 + Ipamorelin encourages your own growth hormone pulse to return toward youthful, which often translates to better recovery, deeper sleep, fat loss, and more satisfying training. Tesamorelin focuses specifically on reducing visceral fat while preserving muscle. Sermorelin is a lighter-touch option for the same pathway. BPC-157 tells tissues to mend—gut lining, tendons, ligaments, and muscle—making it especially helpful when inflammation or injury has kept you on the sidelines. KPV is a potent anti-inflammatory messenger, particularly for the gut and skin. PT-141 acts centrally on the brain's arousal pathways and can restore libido in both women and men independent of testosterone levels. GHK-Cu is a copper peptide long valued for skin and hair quality—useful when hormonal changes make you look older than you feel. MOTS-C with AICAR targets the mitochondria that power your cells, improving endurance, glucose handling, and overall energy output. None of these replaces hormones; they amplify your body's response once the hormonal baseline is set.

Nutraceuticals supply the raw materials and stabilizers that keep hormones working as intended. DIM Plus helps metabolize estrogen down safer pathways, which can matter for both men and women when estrogen is high relative to other hormones. ADK10—vitamins A, D3, and K2—supports bone density, vascular health, immune resilience, and hormone receptor sensitivity. Super Omega 3D balances inflammatory signals, supporting the brain, joints, and cardiovascular system. Super B (a methylated B complex) bolsters energy production and methylation, a key detox process that affects hormone balance. Mag Complete brings sleep quality and muscle relaxation back online. Thyroid Complete offers iodine, selenium, zinc, and co-factors that help the thyroid convert T4 to active T3. For gut-immune stability, IgG binds and clears microbial fragments, while targeted protocols like Remove Complete, ParaKill, and

CandiKill—used judiciously and temporarily—can clear overgrowths that keep inflammation high and hormones noisy. The short version: hormones signal, peptides direct, nutraceuticals supply, and lifestyle locks it in.

Lifestyle is the amplifier. Resistance training two to three times a week is not cosmetic—it's hormonal therapy by another name. Muscle is the largest sink for glucose in your body, and it releases anti-inflammatory myokines that talk to your brain and immune system. Daily walking stabilizes blood sugar and cortisol. Sunlight early in the day anchors your circadian rhythm; darkness at night lets melatonin do its job. A protein-forward, colorful, minimally processed diet keeps insulin stable and gives the liver what it needs to process hormones cleanly. Alcohol complicates everything—sleep, estrogen metabolism, cortisol—so shrinking the weekly total often does more for your hormones than any single supplement.

If you want to feel how hormones touch every corner of life, picture three people at different ages. A forty-seven-year-old woman notices her cycle shortening and her patience thinning. She wakes at 3 a.m. several nights a week and dreads presentations she would have breezed through a year ago. Her labs show low progesterone and declining estrogen with low free testosterone. Bringing progesterone back into physiologic range helps her fall and stay asleep; gentle estrogen replacement restores cognitive ease and joint comfort; low-dose testosterone returns her midsection and her momentum. A fifty-six-year-old man feels a quiet flattening of mood and strength, with afternoon slumps, softening muscle, and creeping belly fat. His testosterone is "low-normal," estradiol is too low for joint comfort, DHEA is depleted, and fasting insulin is high. Restoring testosterone, supporting estradiol into range, adding DHEA, and re-training insulin with nutrition and walking bring him back to himself. A sixty-two-year-old woman, years past menopause, fears the aches and fog are permanent. Her bone density scan nudges her toward medications she hopes to avoid. Optimizing estrogen and progesterone, adding ADK10 and omega-3s, training with resistance, and using peptides for recovery shift the trajectory—in her bones, her balance, and her belief that strong is still available.

"Did You Know?" moments help make this real. Estrogen supports synapse formation in the brain, which is one reason many women notice memory lapses when it falls. Progesterone interacts with GABA receptors—the brain's calming system—explaining its effect on peaceful sleep. Testosterone influences dopamine pathways, the chemistry of drive and satisfaction, not just muscle size. Thyroid hormones determine how many mitochondria you build and how energetically they work. Cortisol's curve shapes your appetite, your focus, and your willingness to exercise. When you tune the messengers, you unjam the traffic in your whole life.

A note about quality and sourcing: use licensed providers, legitimate pharmacies, and evidence-based protocols. "More" is not better; "yours" is better. The right dose is the one that returns function without overshooting. Monitor with labs and how you feel. Expect adjustments. Your biology is dynamic, and your plan should be, too.

If you're wondering where to start, start with seeing. Ask for a thorough panel, not just a screening TSH or a single testosterone reading. Look at patterns, not snapshots. Pair those results with your lived experience—sleep, mood, energy, libido, workouts, digestion, skin, hair—and build your plan in a sensible order: restore the signals, provide the materials, remove friction, and reinforce the rhythms. Within weeks, you'll sense alignment. Within months, others will see it. Within a year, your labs will tell a younger story.

This is the hormone connection—less a mystery than a conversation you finally learn to hear. In the next chapter, we'll go deeper into **what BHRT is and isn't**, how it differs from synthetic hormones, what delivery methods exist, how safety is determined, and why personalization is the non-negotiable rule of the road. For now, hold this thought: when your messengers speak clearly, every other effort you make—nutrition, training, sleep, stress work—suddenly works better.

Chapter 3

Understanding BHRT

Bioidentical Hormone Replacement Therapy (BHRT) is the simple idea that when the body's natural messengers get too quiet, we can restore them—carefully, thoughtfully, and in forms the body recognizes—so you can feel and function like yourself again. If Chapter 2 made the case that hormones are the master signals for energy, mood, metabolism, sleep, muscle, and sexual health, this chapter shows how we restore those signals in real life, with a special focus on a delivery method that solves one of the most common problems in hormone care: inconsistency. That method is bioidentical estradiol and testosterone delivered by pellets placed beneath the skin by a trusted provider. Pellets release hormone gently and steadily for months, so you're not chasing highs and lows or forgetting daily doses. For many women and men, this "set-it-and-live-your-life" approach becomes the most sustainable way to regain themselves.

Before we zoom in on pellets, let's ground ourselves in what BHRT actually is, and what it isn't. BHRT uses molecules that are structurally identical to what your body makes—estradiol (E2), estriol (E3), progesterone, testosterone, DHEA, and thyroid hormones (T4 and T3). When these levels drift below the zones where humans tend to feel and perform best, function slips. Sleep lightens. Mood gets brittle. Muscles shrink from the same workouts that used to build them. Belly fat appears without permission. Libido and spontaneous desire fade. Concentration feels like pushing through fog. BHRT restores those messages with precision—aiming for physiologic, youthful ranges, not body-builder peaks—and pairs them with monitoring so your care stays individualized and safe.

Many people hesitate around hormones because of old headlines and half-told stories. A lot of the confusion came from studies that bundled different molecules, different doses, different routes, and different ages into a single bucket and then drew sweeping conclusions. In real life, the safety profile of transdermal bioidentical estradiol plus physiologic progesterone looks different from high-dose oral estrogens paired with non-bioidentical progestins. Timing matters. Route matters. Individualization matters. When done thoughtfully, BHRT is not a reckless experiment; it's a respectful restoration of biology.

Now, about pellets—and why this chapter places them front and center for estradiol and testosterone. A pellet is a tiny cylinder of compressed bioidentical hormone placed just under the skin—usually in the upper outer buttock or hip area—during a brief office procedure under local anesthetic. Once in place, the pellet dissolves slowly and releases hormone at a stable rate into the bloodstream, creating an even hormonal "background" that feels natural and requires no daily action from you. Most women need re-insertion about every 3–4 months and most men about every 4–6 months, depending on dose, metabolism, and activity level. The result: consistent levels, consistent days, and a chance for the rest of your plan—nutrition, training, sleep—to work without sabotage from fluctuating signals.

Why does this matter so much? Because consistency is everything with hormones. Many people starting with creams or gels do fine at first, but daily absorption can vary with skin temperature, sweat, shower timing, and application technique. It's common to have "good days and off days" for reasons that have nothing to do with you—just variable uptake. Injections can work beautifully too, but depending on the interval, some people experience peaks and troughs—a few days of feeling amazing followed by a slide before the next dose. Pellets are different. By creating a slow, physiologic trickle, pellets flatten the peaks and fill the valleys, so you feel like the same person on Monday as you do on Thursday and Sunday. For many, that steadiness translates into steadier mood, deeper sleep, more predictable sexual desire, better gym performance, and less "white-knuckling" through the week.

Did You Know? The number one reason people fall off traditional hormone therapy isn't side effects—it's friction. Daily applications, midweek shot scheduling, traveling with supplies, and remembering refills all add up. Pellets compress the task of hormone replacement into a few minutes every several months—and the body handles the rest.

None of this means pellets are magic or "one size fits all." They still need to be individualized. Your dose is calculated based on your baseline labs, symptoms, body composition, activity level, and goals. Your response is monitored with follow-up labs and how you feel. Adjustments are expected in the first one or two cycles while your tissues relearn a youthful signal. A trusted provider experienced with pellets is essential—technique matters, insertion matters, dose titration matters, and follow-up matters.

Let's anchor this in real lives. Ava was fifty, a project director who couldn't remember the last time she slept straight through the night. Her cycles had gone erratic, her patience felt thin, and her body composition had shifted in ways she didn't recognize. She had tried a topical estrogen and a tiny dose of testosterone cream but felt up-and-down and often forgot applications. On evaluation, her estradiol and progesterone were both low; her free testosterone was barely measurable; and her DHEA had drifted down after years of stress. She chose a pellet-forward plan for estradiol and testosterone, paired with nighttime oral bioidentical progesterone for sleep and uterine protection. Two weeks after insertion she felt a first click: hot flashes calmed and sleep consolidated. At eight weeks, she noticed she was laughing more easily, building muscle again, and saying yes to intimacy for the first time in months. At four months, she returned for re-insertion before levels dipped—no crash, no drama, just continuity.

Pellet therapy doesn't just flatten the peaks and troughs; it also improves adherence. Ask anyone who has tried to keep up with daily creams through a humid summer or a chaotic travel season, or who struggles with injection timing aboard frequent flights. When life is full, the treatment with the least daily friction often wins. That's why pellets are college kid-proof, business-trip-proof, and toddler-bath-time-proof. The hormone signal stays stable regardless of your calendar.

At this point, it's natural to ask, "Is pellet therapy safe?" Safety isn't a yes/no; it's a set of choices that minimize risk while maximizing benefit. With estradiol, route matters for clot risk. Oral estrogens interact with the liver first; transdermal and pellet routes bypass first-pass metabolism. That difference along with right-sized dosing and co-administration of physiologic progesterone when a uterus is present shapes safety in a favorable direction for many women. With testosterone, men and women alike do best when kept in physiologic ranges appropriate to sex and life stage; overshooting is not the goal. Experienced providers are deliberate about starting doses, about letting estradiol in men rise into a comfortable band for joints, libido, and vascular health, and about monitoring hematocrit so blood viscosity stays in a safe zone.

Did You Know? Many women assume testosterone is a "male" hormone and avoid it. In reality, women make and need testosterone—much less than men, but enough that the right level can transform energy, focus, sexual desire, muscle maintenance, and midsection leanness. Pellets allow you to live in that "just right" zone without chasing a rollercoaster.

Let's talk mechanics. A pellet insertion appointment typically takes less than fifteen minutes. The skin is numbed with a local anesthetic. A tiny incision is made—often no longer than a grain of rice—and a trocar places the pellets into the subcutaneous tissue. Two or three steri-strips and a pressure dressing go on top. Aftercare is simple: keep the area dry for the first day, avoid submersion and high-intensity lower-body work for a few days, and then forget about it. Within two weeks most people notice the first shift; within six to eight weeks the full rhythm takes hold. Most women re-insert at 3–4 months; most men at 4–6 months. Some highly active people or those with faster metabolism need slightly earlier re-insertions—your provider will help you find your pattern.

So where do progesterone, DHEA, and thyroid fit into a pellet-forward plan? Progesterone is usually given orally at bedtime in a bioidentical micronized form. Many women describe it as the "exhale" their nervous system was missing: calmer evenings, deeper sleep, fewer nocturnal wake-and-worry trips. DHEA can be replaced in low oral doses when stress and age have depleted it; it quietly supports libido, immunity, and resilience. Thyroid is its own conversation—some people make plenty of T4 but struggle to convert it to T3, the active hormone. In those cases, adding a touch of T3 or improving the "conversion environment" (iron, selenium, zinc, iodine where appropriate; less inflammation; better sleep) can unlock energy and mood.

Case story: Miguel was fifty-six, a small-business owner whose days were long and whose energy was short. He had tried weekly testosterone injections from a friend's gym regimen, felt great for two days, then irritable and flat by day five. His labs showed a "low-normal" total testosterone and very low free testosterone, with estradiol so low his knees ached when he climbed stairs. We moved him to pellet therapy to smooth the curve and let estradiol rise into a comfortable, joint-protective band through aromatization. He added two short strength workouts per week and daily walks. At six weeks, he noticed he woke up before his alarm; at three months, he could climb stairs without knee complaints and had dropped his afternoon energy slump. He now re-inserts every five months to avoid a dip at the end of cycle.

Pellets are not only about convenience and steadiness; they also support a bigger project: rebuilding capacity. When hormones are steady, sleep consolidates. When sleep consolidates, your brain clears waste better, your insulin sensitivity improves, and your cravings quiet. When cravings quiet, you can choose food that supports hormone metabolism—protein-forward, colorful, minimally processed meals that your body reads as "safe to burn, safe to repair." When your energy is even, you train with traction and recover faster, which protects and builds the muscle that acts like a longevity organ. And because pellets are not a daily task, your bandwidth is free to focus on the habits that compound.

Did You Know? Skeletal muscle is the largest glucose sink in the body. Steadier testosterone and estradiol support the muscle you have and the muscle you're building—one reason strength training plus pellet-based BHRT is such a powerful longevity duo.

Let's get practical about testing and monitoring with a pellet-forward plan. Before your first insertion, you and your provider should have a full picture: estradiol (sensitive assay), progesterone (if cycling, timed appropriately), total and free testosterone, DHEA-S, SHBG, a complete thyroid panel (TSH, free T4, free T3, reverse T3, antibodies when appropriate), and metabolic markers like fasting insulin and glucose, A1C, lipids with particle information when available, inflammatory markers such as hs-CRP, ferritin, vitamin D, B12/folate, homocysteine, and a basic chemistry panel. If you're a man, include hematocrit/hemoglobin and PSA as clinically indicated. If you're a woman with a uterus, ensure progesterone coverage is in place when estradiol is restored. Re-check labs at 6–8 weeks after initial insertion to confirm trajectory, again around 3–4 months (or just before your next insertion), and then settle into a rhythm that matches your cycle—often 3–6 months during the first year, then semiannual or annual once stable.

Because this chapter is pellet-forward, it's worth briefly comparing the pharmacologic feel of different delivery routes so you can appreciate why the "texture" of your days changes. Topical creams and gels can deliver steady levels when applied consistently, but absorption varies from person to person and even day to day with skin hydration, sweat, and temperature. Injections deliver a known dose on a schedule; some people prefer a higher-frequency micro-dosing schedule to reduce peaks and troughs, and that can work very well. Pellets minimize user error and day-to-day variability by design. The best route is the one that (1) gives you stable physiology, (2) fits your life, and (3) you can actually sustain. For many busy adults, pellets check those boxes more easily than anything else.

What about side effects? The most common with pellets are local and short-lived: bruising, mild soreness, or a small temporary bump at the insertion site that softens as the pellet dissolves. Systemic effects are dose-related and fixable with adjustments. In women, if testosterone overshoots, you might notice oily skin or acne or hair changes; that's a signal to nudge the dose down, not a reason to abandon therapy. In men, if hematocrit rises or blood feels "thick," plan a donation and a dose review. If estradiol is too low in men, joints can ache and libido can fall; if too high, fluid retention or breast tenderness can occur—both are addressed by dose, interval, and lifestyle. Working with a provider who follows you closely makes these tweaks straightforward.

Nutrition, detoxification, and the gut matter more than most people realize when hormones change. Your gut and liver co-author your hormone story. If the gut is inflamed, estrogen can recirculate in forms you don't want; if the liver is overburdened, thyroid conversion stalls and fatigue lingers. This is where targeted nutraceuticals help the body receive hormone signals cleanly. A methylated B-complex (Super B) supports energy production and methylation pathways needed for hormone metabolism. Vitamins A, D3, and K2 (ADK10) help maintain bone density, immune balance, and hormone receptor sensitivity. Omega-3s in balanced EPA/DHA forms (Super Omega 3D) reduce inflammatory "noise" so signals land. Magnesium (Mag Complete) smooths sleep and muscle tension. For estrogen metabolism specifically, diindolylmethane complexes (DIM Plus) help steer estrogen down safer pathways. If the gut needs repair, immunoglobulins (IgG), gut-soothing blends (GI-support formulas), and targeted antimicrobials when appropriate (programs akin to Remove Complete, ParaKill, or CandiKill) can help re-establish balance so nutrients absorb and hormones metabolize.

Pellets play particularly well with peptides because the steady hormone signal creates an ideal background for cellular repair. Growth hormone secretagogues such as CJC-1295 + Ipamorelin often deepen sleep and speed recovery from training; with steady testosterone and estradiol on board, that recovery goes somewhere meaningful—toward stronger connective tissue, better body composition, and richer mornings. Tesamorelin can help reduce visceral fat while preserving muscle. Sermorelin is a gentler nudge to the same pathway. BPC-157 supports tendon, ligament, muscle, and gut healing. TB500 can reduce friction in inflamed or overused areas. KPV calms inflammatory signaling in the gut and systemically. MOTS-C + AICAR supports mitochondrial efficiency, making energy production feel smoother. Used in cycles with monitoring, these peptides complement pellet-based BHRT beautifully.

Case story: Priya, forty-seven, had tried to white-knuckle her way through perimenopause. She ran five miles three times a week and skipped breakfast, hoping her body would get the message. It didn't. Sleep was broken, weight crept upward, and her fuse was short with the people she loved most. On labs, estradiol was low for her age, progesterone was barely measurable, and free testosterone was almost absent. We chose a pellet-forward plan for estradiol and testosterone with nighttime progesterone, layered in CJC-1295 + Ipamorelin for 12 weeks to deepen sleep and amplify recovery, and tuned her nutrition toward protein-forward, colorful, minimally processed meals. At three months she said, "I didn't know it could be this quiet inside my head." At nine months, she was lifting with enjoyment, sleeping through, and described her marriage as "easier, because I feel like me."

A pellet-forward plan still respects individuality. Some people do best beginning with slightly smaller pellet doses and stepping up over the first year; others need a stronger first placement and then a lower maintenance dose. Some women prefer to keep estradiol a touch lower and testosterone a touch higher for libido and energy; others want the opposite for joint comfort and sleep depth. Some men prefer re-insertion at five months instead of six to avoid even a mild end-cycle dip. The point is not to copy a protocol; it's to build your protocol.

Did You Know? The lab range called "normal" is a statistical snapshot of the population—not a performance target. Many midlife adults sit inside "normal" ranges while feeling unwell. In practice, "optimal" is where you sleep, think, move, recover, and connect like yourself again.

You might be wondering when you'll notice changes. Progesterone's effect on sleep is often felt within days. Estradiol shifts build over weeks as tissues regain elasticity and thermoregulation steadies. Testosterone's benefits accrue with time as muscles receive and respond to the "build and repair" message; many people report clearer morning energy and stronger workouts by week four to six. Bone density and body composition are slower, month-to-year projects—but they are precisely the projects that determine whether your 70s and 80s feel like an extension of your prime or a struggle for independence. Steady pellets support those long arcs.

Let's address common myths, pellet-forward. "Once you start hormones, your body stops making them." By the time most people consider BHRT, their endogenous production has already declined; BHRT restores signals you no longer produce in adequate amounts. "Pellets are permanent." Pellets dissolve; their effect tapers naturally, which is why you return every four to six months. "Pellets give everyone acne or hair changes." Those effects are dose-related and uncommon when female targets are respected, and men are monitored. "Pellets are only for people who don't want to do the work." The opposite is true: pellets remove daily friction so your work—nutrition, training, sleep, stress skills—actually sticks.

A word about quality and sourcing. Use licensed, reputable pharmacies and clinicians who do a lot of insertions and follow their patients closely. Technique matters for comfort and for minimizing local issues. Dose calculation tools exist, but experience still counts when translating a number into a human day. Be wary of "more is better." The right dose is the smallest dose that returns you to function and well-being without overshooting. Monitor with labs and with your life: sleep, mood, sex drive, recovery, appetite, and focus.

Pellet therapy does not replace the foundations that make hormone messages land. Protein-forward meals tell your body it is safe to repair and build. Colorful plants provide fiber and phytochemicals that support estrogen metabolism and gut health. Healthy fats—olive oil, avocado, nuts, egg yolks—fortify cell membranes and act as the raw material for steroid hormones. Strength training two to three days a week protects muscle and bone; daily walking stabilizes insulin and calms your nervous system. Morning light anchors circadian rhythm; darkness at night lets melatonin work. Magnesium in the evening, omega-3s with the first meal, ADK10 regularly, and DIM Plus as needed are simple anchors that compound.

Case story: Daniel, sixty-one, had retired early and expected to feel free. Instead, he felt flat. He forgot names. He skipped golf because he was tired. His wife saw the light go out behind his eyes. His labs read like a common midlife pattern: low free testosterone, estradiol too low for joint comfort, vitamin D low, A1C creeping up. Pellet therapy gave him back a stable floor under his days. He began to lift twice weekly, walked after dinner, added protein at breakfast, and took omega-3s and magnesium consistently. At his six-month visit, he said, "I feel like my life fits me again."

So—why lead with pellets in a book about BHRT? Because for many adults who want to live fully without micromanaging their therapy, pellets solve the day-to-day problems: they remove user error, smooth variability, and free you to build a life around stable energy, mood, and desire. They do not have to be your forever route; you can change later if life changes. But for a huge number of people—busy parents, traveling professionals, caretakers, anyone who wants fewer decisions each week—pellets are the route that keeps the main thing the main thing: living.

Practical FAQ

- How long do pellets last? Most women re-insert about every 3–4 months; most men every 4–6 months. Your interval is individualized.
- Does it hurt? It's quick, with local anesthetic. Mild soreness or bruising is possible for a few days.
- Will I feel "not myself"? The goal is the opposite: to restore you to yourself. Doses target physiologic ranges, not extremes.
- What about fertility? Men who plan to conceive soon should discuss adjuncts or alternatives (e.g., hCG) because exogenous testosterone suppresses sperm production. Women should discuss contraception separately; pellets are not birth control.
- What if I don't like it? Pellets dissolve gradually. If a dose ever feels too strong, your provider can extend your interval and adjust next time.
- Is it expensive? Consider the cost of doing nothing: lost productivity, low mood, poor sleep, more medications. Pellets often replace other costs by giving you a foundation that makes lifestyle work.

As we close this chapter, remember that a pellet is not the point. The point is what a steady message allows: deep sleep that shows up without pleading, mornings that begin on green instead of red, workouts that reward your effort, intimacy that feels spontaneous again, patience that returns to conversations, and a body composition that moves back toward the shape of your life. BHRT is not an escape from aging; it is a respectful partnership with your biology so you can age like someone with plans.

In the next chapter, we'll translate principles into targets. You'll learn why "normal" lab ranges can be misleading, how "optimal" differs by sex and stage of life, where real-world target zones often live for estradiol, progesterone, testosterone, thyroid, and DHEA, and how pellet-steady signals help you reach and maintain those zones. You'll also see how to pair labs with lived experience so your plan feels personal—not theoretical. For now, hold this truth close: you don't need perfect biology to live well; you need clear signals, steady inputs, and a plan you can sustain.

Chapter 4

The Science of Optimal Hormone Ranges

If you have ever been told that your lab results are "normal" while you feel anything but, you've already met the core problem this chapter solves. Most reference ranges are not maps to true wellness. They are statistical snapshots of the people who happen to get bloodwork at a given lab in a given year, smoothed into a bell curve and trimmed at the edges. That means "normal" often reflects a population with poor sleep, chronic stress, little sunlight, processed diets, and drifting hormones. When you compare yourself to that average, being "normal" can mean fatigued, foggy, anxious, inflamed, and slowly losing muscle and motivation. Optimal is different. Optimal is where your brain is clear, your mood is stable, your energy lasts through the day, your body composition trends leaner, your sex life is alive, your recovery works, and your labs reflect balance instead of compensation. This chapter is about finding that zone—safely, intelligently, and personally—so the rest of your plan finally works.

To understand why optimal matters, think about how hormones signal. Hormones are not just numbers on a report; they are biochemical messages touching nearly every cell. Testosterone influences protein synthesis, red blood cell production, mitochondrial function, and drive in both men and women. Estradiol supports neuronal growth, synaptic plasticity, bone turnover, vascular flexibility, and collagen integrity. Progesterone calms the brain, stabilizes sleep architecture, and balances estrogen's growth signals. Thyroid hormones set the pace for cellular energy. DHEA intersects with immune tone and stress resilience. Cortisol follows a daily rhythm that keeps you alert in the morning and lets you sleep at night. The effect you feel is not just the amount circulating in your blood but whether those signals arrive in the right pattern, at the right time of day, and in a body whose receptors are ready to respond. The difference between "normal" and "optimal" lives in that pattern and responsiveness.

This is why one person with a mid-range testosterone may feel slow and unmotivated, while another at the same number feels fantastic. It isn't only the number; it's binding proteins, receptor sensitivity, micronutrient sufficiency, sleep debt, inflammation, gut health, and mitochondrial capacity. Sex hormone–binding globulin can trap hormones in circulation and make a "normal" total look robust while free and bioavailable fractions are underpowered. Thyroid can look "fine" by TSH alone while free T3 is flat and reverse T3 is high from chronic stress or calorie restriction. Estradiol can be measured with an assay too blunt to detect true levels in women or men, obscuring what's really happening. Cortisol can appear acceptable on a single morning draw even when the 24-hour rhythm is inverted. "Normal" hides in averages. "Optimal" emerges when you layer the right tests, the right timing, and the right context.

The right testing rhythm matters as much as what you test. Hormones are pulsatile. Growth hormone rises in sleep and post-exercise bursts. Cortisol peaks in the morning and should taper smoothly through the day. Estradiol moves across the menstrual cycle, and progesterone rises only after ovulation, so a single random snapshot can look "low" or "high" without meaning anything at all. Testosterone can be transiently suppressed by sleep loss, alcohol, acute illness, or a heavy endurance block, then rebound within days or weeks once recovery is restored. Because the body speaks in rhythms, we listen in rhythms. That means drawing sex hormones first thing in the morning, repeating them when symptoms and context suggest a change, tracking thyroid with free fractions and reverse T3 when energy, weight, or temperature regulation stall, and assessing cortisol across the day when sleep or stress is off. If you measure the wrong time or the wrong fraction, you can talk yourself into a false story about your biology.

It helps to imagine a series of concentric circles. At the center are your lived symptoms: energy, mood, sleep quality, libido, strength gains, recovery, body composition, menstrual regularity or menopausal comfort, and cognitive clarity. Around that sits a circle of core labs: for sex hormones, total and free testosterone, estradiol by a reliable method, progesterone timed appropriately; for thyroid, TSH with free T4, free T3, and reverse T3; for adrenal rhythm, morning cortisol with context or a diurnal profile when needed; and for metabolic health, fasting insulin, A1c, a meaningful lipid picture, hs-CRP, ferritin, vitamin D, B12 or methylmalonic acid, and homocysteine. The outer circle holds the terrain: micronutrients such as zinc, selenium, iodine when appropriate, magnesium, and omega-3 status; the state of the gut barrier and microbiome; sleep timing and consistency; training load and recovery; and the environmental stressors you carry. When all three circles are reviewed together, the numbers start to make sense, and the plan becomes obvious.

For women, optimal is a moving target if you only chase numbers, because the physiology moves by design. In the reproductive years, estradiol rises before ovulation and progesterone anchors the luteal phase; both have brain and bone benefits that extend far beyond reproduction. Testosterone is made by the ovaries and adrenals and is critical for muscle, motivation, and libido, even if the absolute number is much lower than in men. The goal is not to pin estradiol or progesterone to a single line on a graph; it is to restore the pattern that produces steady energy, deep sleep, stable mood, midsection calm instead of bloat, comfortable cycles, and a sex drive that feels like you. As women transition into perimenopause, the pattern becomes erratic, and symptoms—not just lab snapshots—become the compass. This is where individualized bioidentical hormone replacement can reclaim quality of life, not by forcing youthful extremes, but by restoring a physiologic signal that the body recognizes.

In menopause, estradiol and progesterone fall and stay low without support, and the costs show up in joint stiffness, brain fog, mood lability, dry tissues, and bone loss over time. Here, "optimal" means symptoms recede, sleep normalizes, cognition steadies, and markers of bone and cardiovascular health move in the right direction, using the lowest effective doses adjusted patiently over months. Testosterone support in women is equally about function. The aim is not a number on paper but a return of motivation, strength, and sexual wellbeing without side effects. The right approach will feel subtly right within weeks and build steadily over months. If it does not, the plan can be tuned—delivery route, dose, interval, and the nutritional and lifestyle factors that make receptors responsive.

For men, the myth is that testosterone inexorably falls and there is nothing you can do. The truth is that testosterone is sensitive to sleep, stress, central adiposity, alcohol intake, micronutrient status, thyroid function, and inflammatory burden. "Normal" male ranges are wide, and many men feel underpowered when they sit at the low end. Again, free testosterone, not just total, is where the signal lands. Men with high SHBG can feel flat with a middle-of-the-road total because free is low. Men with low SHBG can look low-normal total while free is acceptable. The aim is not to chase supra-physiologic numbers; it is to restore a physiologic strength of signal that translates into steady morning energy, reliable workouts, faster recovery, healthy body composition, stable mood, and a sex life that feels natural. If those don't appear, the solution isn't automatically "more." It may be better sleep, less alcohol, more protein, a change in delivery route, a correction in thyroid, a reduction in evening stressors that flatten the morning cortisol rise, or targeted support that improves receptor sensitivity.

Thyroid deserves special attention because it multiplies every other signal. Thyroid hormones sit upstream of oxygen consumption, heat production, and mitochondrial turnover. You can be "normal" by TSH but still feel slow if free T3 is low from chronic stress, low calorie intake, inflammatory cytokines, or micronutrient gaps. Optimal thyroid function shows up as consistent energy across the day, comfortable body temperature, a heart rate that matches your level of fitness rather than the tension in your life, hair and skin that hold their quality, and a metabolism that responds to reasonable nutrition and training. A plan for thyroid is not just about replacing hormone when needed; it is also about supplying iodine judiciously, ensuring selenium for conversion and redox balance, zinc for receptor function, magnesium for enzymatic work, iron sufficiency for thyroid peroxidase, and vitamin D for immune balance. When those ingredients are present, a modest dose can go further and the right dose becomes clear.

Cortisol is neither villain nor hero; it is the rhythm that sets you up for the day. The optimal pattern is a crisp rise in the morning, a calm, gradually declining curve through the afternoon, and a low, sleepy trough at night. When the curve flattens, mornings feel like slog, cravings increase, and late-day energy can be wired or brittle. When the signal spikes at night, sleep fractures. Restoring optimal here is not about obliterating cortisol; it is about restoring its timing. Morning daylight outside, consistent wake times, and movement shortly after breakfast create a powerful anchor. A protein-forward breakfast dampens mid-morning cravings. Evening light hygiene, a cooler bedroom, and a calming wind-down routine lower the curve at night. If stress physiology has been stretched thin for years, targeted support can help rebuild the curve. Ingredients such as B-vitamins in methylated forms, magnesium glycinate or taurate, omega-3 fatty acids, and adaptogens that cushion the stress response without sedation are practical tools. When cortisol timing improves, sex hormones and thyroid often follow suit because the stress signal is no longer demanding center stage.

All of these signals sit inside a terrain. Receptor sensitivity rises when the membrane is healthy, and that depends on fatty acid balance, micronutrients, and inflammation control. It is not a coincidence that so many people feel "hormone resistant" when their diet leans on refined grains and industrial oils. Those inputs build fragile membranes, generate oxidative stress, and command your hormonal system to fight fires rather than rebuild. Replacing that pattern with clean proteins, colorful plants rich in polyphenols, and natural fats like olive oil, avocado, pasture-raised egg yolks, and a meaningful intake of omega-3s turns the terrain from reactive to responsive. When the terrain improves, smaller hormonal adjustments create bigger results.

This is where targeted nutraceuticals quietly change the game. When the daily diet covers the basics but modern life leaves gaps, supplementation supplies the missing co-factors that let hormones work. A methylated B complex supports methylation cycles involved in neurotransmitter balance and steroid hormone metabolism, while noticeable effects include steadier energy, fewer afternoon slumps, and better resilience under cognitive load. A thoughtful fat-soluble trio of vitamins A, D3, and K2 supports hormone receptor signaling, bone metabolism, and vascular flexibility, which shows up as steadier blood pressure tendencies, stronger bones over serial scans, and fewer soft-tissue aches as collagen tissue quality rises. High-quality fish-derived omega-3s with adequate potency reduce inflammatory tone, soften joint discomfort, support brain function, and tend to improve triglyceride and lipoprotein patterns. For people with sluggish thyroid physiology or a history of dieting, a blend that supplies iodine, selenium, zinc, and other co-factors gives the enzyme systems what they were missing; when thyroid replacement is warranted, those nutrients make the dose work better. Magnesium in a chelated form helps muscles relax at night, reduces tension headaches, eases restless legs, and deepens sleep. Coenzyme Q10 supports mitochondrial ATP production in high-demand tissues like the heart, brain, and active muscle; when combined with dimethylglycine, the effect during submaximal exertion can feel like the engine runs cooler at the same speed, with fewer post-exertional slumps. None of these are hormones, yet they make hormones act as if the volume knob is finally connected to the speakers.

If estrogen metabolism is on your mind—especially for women using bioidentical estradiol or navigating perimenopause—dietary cruciferous vegetables and specific nutritional support can encourage healthier pathways, shifting phase I and phase II metabolism toward gentler metabolites and consistent clearance. The real-world effect feels like less bloat, steadier mood, clearer skin, and more predictable cycles or symptom control. If the gut is inflamed or porous, immune traffic rises, and the hormonal system hears it as a stressor. Helping the gut barrier and immune balance with targeted immunoglobulins, soothing nutrients for the intestinal lining, and a remove-repair-reseed progression breaks the loop. When the gut quiets, the skin often follows, cravings calm, sleep improves, and hormone adjustments land cleanly instead of ricocheting.

Peptides are not a replacement for hormones or nutrition; they are signal boosters you can point where you need them. When growth hormone pulses are anemic from age, stress, or sleep debt, carefully cycling a combination that nudges your own nightly pulses can improve body composition and recovery, especially when you're lifting and eating sufficient protein. When injuries or inflamed tendons are the bottleneck, healing peptides that signal repair at the capillary and fibroblast level help you get back to the strength training that protects bone and muscle—and therefore protects your long-term hormone needs. When brain energy is the limiter, a stack that emphasizes cellular energy and synaptic plasticity makes cognitive tasks feel more fluid, which is often what people mean when they say their "hormones finally kicked in." The important point is that peptides are most effective when the rest of the plan already respects circadian biology, protein intake, and sleep. They are multipliers, not substitutes.

"Optimal" is not a one-time achievement; it is a moving conversation between your goals and your biology. When someone starts bioidentical hormone replacement, the first wins often arrive as better sleep and less mental noise. Body composition follows as training and nutrition stabilize. Libido returns once the nervous system stops bracing and starts trusting again. Those early gains are real, but the full picture emerges over three to six months as receptors adjust, tissues remodel, and your daily habits support the new set point. The smartest thing you can do during that time is to keep the rest of your life predictable enough to learn what works. Pick a bedtime window and defend it. Anchor your morning with light and protein. Strength train two to four days a week, focusing on compound movements and progressive overload. Walk after meals. Keep alcohol modest. Get outside. Put your phone down an hour before bed. These ordinary behaviors do extraordinary things for hormone signaling. They are the difference between "numbers look better" and "my life feels better."

Lab follow-up should match physiology, not a calendar on the wall. Early in a new plan, check in with your symptoms every week and repeat targeted labs every six to twelve weeks, not to chase perfection but to confirm direction. If your plan includes a delivery route that yields steady levels over months, you can push lab intervals longer once your symptoms and training data are stable. When something changes in the rest of your life—major stress, travel, sleep disruption, illness—be patient with your body and hold major dose changes until the dust settles. Hormones are not meant to be jerked around by your calendar; they are meant to be tuned.

It is helpful to think about ranges as a neighborhood rather than a single address. There is usually a low side where symptoms creep in and a high side where diminishing returns or side effects appear. The optimal window for you is where your day feels effortless more often, where your training feels productive rather than punitive, and where recovery happens during sleep instead of stealing it. That window may shift as you lose visceral fat, as your muscle mass grows, as your job changes, or as you move through perimenopause into menopause or through midlife into later decades. Don't be surprised when optimal at 42 is not exactly optimal at 58. Be pleased that you know how to find it again.

One of the reasons the "normal vs. optimal" debate gets heated is that people assume optimal means extreme. It does not. Optimal is often modest-to-upper-middle within a physiologic window, delivered in a way that your body recognizes, and supported by daily behaviors that make receptors responsive and inflammation low. People get into trouble when they mistake stimulation for restoration, over-relying on caffeine and pre-workouts to manufacture energy instead of building it with sleep and protein, or when they push doses looking for shortcuts while leaving the basics undone. Nothing ages a body faster than asking it to sprint without breakfast, sleep, or micronutrients. Nothing creates sustainable momentum faster than doing the simple things at the right time, then layering precise therapy on top.

It's also worth recognizing the psychological shift that happens when you stop chasing "normal." Many people have internalized the idea that fatigue, low motivation, and weight gain are personal failures. When labs finally reflect a plan that supports you, there is often a sense of relief: the engine isn't broken; it was running on the wrong fuel with a misaligned timing belt. That shift matters because it changes how you show up for the plan. You stop bargaining with yourself and start behaving like an athlete in training for the sport of your life.

Another practical truth is that your muscle is the ally of every hormone. Skeletal muscle does more than move weight; it stores glucose safely, disposes of insulin, secretes anti-inflammatory myokines, and communicates with your brain. If your muscle mass is inadequate, hormones have fewer places to dock their benefits. Strength training three days a week is not optional if you want your hormone plan to work; it is the amplifier. Combined with protein at each meal, creatine if you tolerate it, omega-3s to reduce joint friction, and magnesium at night, lifting turns a flat hormonal symphony into music. In older adults, the difference is the difference between independence and frailty. In younger adults, it is the difference between a body that looks like it works and a body that actually works.

You can measure progress in more ways than a lab portal. Track how fast you fall asleep and how often you wake. Track morning energy before caffeine. Track your pull-ups, push-ups, and a simple lift like the deadlift, even if you start with a kettlebell. Track a twenty-minute brisk walk after dinner and how your sleep changes. Track waist circumference at the level of your belly button, not because of vanity but because visceral fat is a hormone-disrupting organ and shrinking it unlocks better signaling. Track resting heart rate and variability, not to obsess over numbers but to notice when stress is accumulating and you need an earlier bedtime, an easier training day, or a little more daylight and less screen light. Track how often you laugh. Track whether you say yes to invitations again. Biology is personal, and so are the metrics that matter.

You may be wondering where safety fits into optimal ranges. Safety begins with bioidentical molecules—signals your body knows how to read—and continues with dose, delivery, and follow-up that reflect your biology rather than an average. Safety is also built by supplying raw materials. Fat-soluble vitamins in balance support bone and cardiovascular integrity when sex hormones are restored. Omega-3s help resolve inflammatory whispers that otherwise become shouts. B-vitamins keep methylation and neurotransmitter pathways moving in the background so you sleep instead of ruminate. Magnesium lets the nervous system and muscles exhale. Coenzyme Q10 and dimethylglycine support mitochondrial work so you can translate hormone signals into real energy. When those pieces are in place, doses do less heavy lifting and side effects are less likely because you are not asking hormones to fix deficits they were never designed to fix.

There will always be marketing promising shortcuts—foods that pretend to be food, supplements that promise miracles without basics, devices that offer energy while you scroll yourself to midnight. Remember that your biology is still human biology. It wants light in the morning, darkness at night, movement across the day, real protein, real plants, quality fats, clean water, a manageable stress load, and a good reason to get out of bed. It appreciates therapy that respects physiology and it rejects therapy that ignores it. The reason the same hormone program produces different results in different people is not luck; it is terrain. Build the terrain, and modest therapy works like magic.

There is an old idea that aging is a story of inevitable decline. The more we measure, the more we see that aging is also a story of adaptability. People in their fifties and sixties routinely outlift and outthink their forties once their hormones are tuned, their sleep is restored, and their training and nutrition match their goals. Women who feared they had to accept hot flashes, insomnia, and diminished desire as the new normal live decades with none of that once they are properly supported. Men who thought they had lost their edge discover it was hiding behind late-night screens, skipped meals, and a cortisol curve stuck in reverse. None of this requires perfection. It requires an honest view of your inputs and a plan to stack them in your favor.

If there is a single sentence to carry from this chapter, let it be this: normal is a statistic; optimal is how you live. You do not need to choose between numbers and feelings. You can have both—labs that reflect health and a life that feels like yours again. The path there is neither mysterious nor extreme. Test what matters, at the right times, with the right methods. Read labs through the lens of symptoms and terrain. Restore signals with bioidentical hormones when appropriate. Use peptides to accelerate repair where you need it. Supply the missing nutrients so the signals land. Guard your sleep like a priceless tool. Train your muscles as if your future depends on them, because it does. Eat food that looks like it grew somewhere. Go outside. Laugh with people you love. Review, adjust, and keep moving.

Did you know that a meaningful share of what we call "hormone resistance" is actually circadian disruption and nutrient insufficiency standing in the way of receptor function? When people restore morning light and protein, move after meals, take in adequate omega-3s and magnesium, and give themselves a dark, cool, quiet bedroom, their "resistance" often melts to response—without changing the dose. That isn't magic; it is physiology reclaiming its rhythm. It is also why a chapter on ranges has turned out to be a chapter on living. Numbers matter, but what you do with them matters more.

When you and your clinician talk about targets, speak in outcomes. "I want energy that lasts until evening without relying on caffeine." "I want to wake up ready to move." "I want my workouts to build me up instead of take me down." "I want a sex life that feels natural again." "I want to remember names and where I put my keys." "I want to feel calm in my own skin." Labs are tools to get you there. They are not grades. They are not judgments. They are glimpses of a living system that responds better than most people have been led to believe. If there is a through-line in every transformation you will read in this book, it is that people stop outsourcing their biology to averages. They become participants. They learn to see patterns. They make small, consistent changes. They measure wisely. They iterate with a steady hand. And then, almost predictably, they become the kind of "outliers" who feel years younger than their birthdays suggest.

That is the promise of optimal ranges—not chasing perfection, but living in a body that responds. When hormones carry clear messages, when receptors are ready, when sleep and nutrition and movement cooperate, life regains momentum. You handle stress better without needing to numb it. You recover faster without needing to skip what you love. You look in the mirror and recognize the person who shows up for the day. None of that is an accident. It is the product of choosing optimal over average, physiology over fashion, and participation over resignation. The science is not a mystery. The art is simply doing it long enough for your biology to believe you.

Chapter 5

The Pellet Advantage: Steady-State Hormones for Real-Life Consistency

The promise of bioidentical hormone replacement therapy (BHRT) is simple: restore the body's own messages so physiology starts working for you again. The challenge is also simple: deliver those messages in a way that is steady, sustainable, and aligned with real life. This chapter focuses on pellet-based BHRT for estradiol and testosterone because, for many people, pellets solve the practical bottlenecks that make other routes hard to live with. But this is not a one-route manifesto. Your hormones, your history, your goals, your schedule—that's the compass. The best route is the one you can live with for years, not weeks.

Why consistency beats intensity. Hormones are not like caffeine or painkillers; you don't want a jolt—you want a background. Your brain, muscles, bones, blood vessels, and sex organs prefer a smooth signal. Fluctuations—big peaks followed by troughs—often feel like mood swings, hot-flash returns, afternoon energy dips, joint discomfort, or libido disappearing and reappearing on a schedule you didn't choose. Pellets release estradiol or testosterone slowly for months, creating a physiological "hum" that most people experience as calmer days, deeper sleep, steadier strength, and more spontaneous intimacy.

How pellets actually work. A pellet is a tiny cylinder of compressed bioidentical hormone placed just under the skin with local anesthetic through a small incision. Once inserted, it dissolves as blood flow and tissue enzymes interact with it, releasing hormone in proportion to your body's demand. Most women return every three to four months and most men every four to six months, though intervals are individualized. After the brief healing period, the pellet simply lives in the background while you live your life in the foreground.

Pharmacokinetics in plain English. Topical creams and gels depend on skin absorption; heat, sweat, shower timing, and application technique introduce daily variability. Patches deliver more consistent estradiol for some users but can irritate skin and peel at inconvenient times. Injections deliver a known quantity on a schedule, but the spacing of shots determines how much you ride a peak-and-valley curve. Oral routes for estradiol engage the liver first, altering clotting proteins and triglycerides, which changes the risk/benefit conversation for some people. Pellets bypass first-pass liver metabolism and flatten the curve across months.

Safety is a pattern, not a headline. The safest plan uses physiologic doses, a route that fits your biology, and real monitoring. For estradiol, non-oral routes reduce first-pass liver effects. For testosterone, steady delivery with oversight protects against issues like excessive hematocrit or overly suppressed estradiol. With pellets, you still monitor labs and symptoms and you still fine-tune dose and interval—especially across the first one or two cycles. Safety grows from personalization and follow-through.

Who tends to thrive on pellets. People who travel, caretakers with unpredictable schedules, high achievers with meeting-packed calendars, and anyone who struggles with remembering daily creams or weekly shots often find pellets liberating. People who feel best on a flat, consistent signal notice fewer mood swings and steadier workouts. And those who want to eliminate the "how am I dosing this week?" decision fatigue appreciate compressing their hormone care into a short appointment every few months.

Who might choose another route. If you are very early in your BHRT journey and want to "tiptoe in," a rapidly adjustable method (topical or injection) can help you find your target before you move to pellets. If you have a history of difficult wound healing or you're in the middle of marathon training that makes post-procedure restrictions hard to honor for a few days, timing matters. If you are planning conception soon (men), pellets with exogenous testosterone are not a fit; there are alternatives to preserve fertility.

Comparing Pellets to Every Other Route—Estradiol.

Estradiol Pellets: Pellets offer a slow, steady delivery that closely matches the body's preference for a background tone of estrogen. Women commonly report better sleep continuity, fewer thermoregulation swings, and more predictable mood and vaginal tissue comfort. Because pellets bypass the liver, they avoid the first-pass changes to clotting proteins and triglycerides characteristic of some oral estrogens. The main trade-offs: dose adjustments happen at the next insertion (not tomorrow), and insertion requires a brief office procedure with short-term activity modifications.

Estradiol Patches: Patches provide reasonably stable estradiol for some users, are easy to stop or adjust, and avoid first-pass liver effects. Skin sensitivity, adhesive fatigue, or premature peeling can interrupt delivery, and forgetting to replace a patch on time can lead to symptom rebound. For people who tolerate adhesives and maintain a good routine, patches can be a good non-oral option.

Estradiol Gels/Creams: Transdermal gels and creams are convenient and allow fine-tuning, but absorption varies with skin thickness, hydration, ambient temperature, and application site. Some women describe "good days and off days" that track with workouts, sauna use, or seasonal changes. For meticulous daily routines, they work well. For those who want to "dose once and live," pellets reduce the daily variability.

Oral Estradiol: Oral estradiol can be effective for symptom control but engages the liver first, influencing clotting factors and triglycerides and creating a different risk/benefit profile for some women. Dosing is easy to change, which is useful during initial titration. For long-term healthspan goals, many prefer non-oral routes or pellets to minimize hepatic effects while keeping levels consistent.

Estradiol Troches/Sublingual: These bypass portions of first-pass metabolism and are simple to take, but because they are intermittent, some users feel a rise-and-fall within the day. For women who dislike skin products and want non-oral therapy with flexible dosing, troches can be reasonable—just expect to pay attention to timing.

Comparing Pellets to Every Other Route—Testosterone

Testosterone Pellets: Pellets provide a calm, even testosterone signal for months. Men often describe clearer morning drive, stronger training response, more patient mood, and steadier libido without the "two days high, three days low" rollercoaster common with longer injection intervals. Women dosed within physiologic female ranges often notice better midsection leanness, motivation, and sexual satisfaction with fewer application tasks to remember. The trade-offs mirror estradiol pellets: dose changes are made at the next insertion; a brief procedure is required; first two cycles are for fine-tuning.

Testosterone Injections (IM or SubQ): Injections are highly effective and flexible. Shot frequency determines your curve. Weekly or bi-weekly dosing can create noticeable peaks and troughs; more frequent micro-dosing flattens the curve but increases task load. Injections are easy to adjust quickly. For people who enjoy hands-on control and don't mind needles or schedules, injections can be a strong choice. For those who travel or dislike self-injection, pellets remove the friction.

Testosterone Transdermals (Gels/Creams): Daily application is simple and allows small adjustments. Variability in absorption can mean variable symptom control; contact transfer to partners or children is a concern that requires careful application and drying. People who keep stable routines often do well; others tire of the daily compliance burden.

Testosterone Troches/Sublingual: Convenient, fast-acting, and adjustable, but like all intermittent methods, they can deliver a noticeable rise-and-fall within a day. Some find the taste or oral effects limiting. For certain use cases, troches are a practical bridge to pellets once a target dose is known.

Testosterone Oral: Non-c17-alkylated oral options exist but are less commonly used because of variability and hepatic considerations in some formulations. For most long-term plans, non-oral routes dominate.

Procedure, Aftercare, and What to Expect. A pellet insertion visit typically takes under fifteen minutes. After numbing, the clinician places pellets via a tiny incision and applies steri-strips and a pressure dressing. Expect mild soreness or bruising for a few days. Keep the site dry for the first day, avoid submersion and high-intensity lower-body training for several days, and then resume normal life.

Most people notice a lifting of baseline energy and steadier sleep within the first two weeks; body composition and bone density are month-to-year projects, but pellets set the conditions for progress.

Dose and interval tuning without the drama. Your first one or two pellet cycles are a learning period. Because pellets are steady, adjustments happen by changing the number of pellets or the interval between insertions. If you feel a gentle dip before your scheduled re-insertion, shorten the interval slightly next time. If you feel over-amped early in a cycle, lower the initial dose. Once your "sweet spot" is found, the plan often runs on rails for long stretches of time with only seasonal tweaks.

What about side effects? With thoughtful dosing and monitoring, most effects are preventable and reversible. In women, dose-related oily skin or acne signal that testosterone is a touch high and should be nudged down. Rare voice changes are avoided by staying within physiologic ranges. Facial hair changes are handled by dose adjustment and standard cosmetic strategies. In men, rising hematocrit calls for a dose review and sometimes a donation. Very low estradiol can feel as bad as too high—joint pain, low mood, flat libido—so balance, not blockade, is the goal.

Safety and monitoring, pellet edition. Baseline labs typically include estradiol, progesterone (timed when cycling), total and free testosterone, SHBG, DHEA-S, a complete thyroid panel (TSH, free T4, free T3, reverse T3, antibodies when indicated), fasting insulin and glucose, A1C, lipids (with particle info when available), hs-CRP, ferritin, vitamin D, and B12/folate as indicated. Recheck after the first cycle at a steady-state point and again near trough before reinsertion. Women with a uterus require bioidentical progesterone alongside estradiol for endometrial protection.

How pellets play with progesterone, thyroid, and peptides. Pellet-steady estradiol and testosterone create a responsive backdrop for oral micronized progesterone at night—often described as the "exhale" that restores deep, continuous sleep and a calmer evening nervous system. Thyroid optimization pairs well with pellets: with steadier sex hormones, conversion of T4 to T3 often stabilizes as sleep improves and inflammation drops. Peptides complement pellets by accelerating repair and improving the behaviors that keep you in range: CJC-1295 + Ipamorelin to deepen sleep and recovery; BPC-157 and TB500 for musculoskeletal healing; Tesamorelin for visceral fat reduction; MOTS-C + AICAR for mitochondrial output and exercise tolerance; PT-141 for centrally mediated libido support when desire lags behind hormones.

Nutrition and nutraceuticals that make pellets work better. Hormones are a signal; food and nutrients are the building materials and the construction crew. A protein-forward pattern with colorful plants and healthy fats gives the body what it needs to respond to estradiol and testosterone. Specific supports often used during BHRT include a methylated B-complex for methylation and energy, vitamins A, D3, and K2 for bone and receptor support, omega-3s for inflammation and vascular health, magnesium for sleep and muscle function, DIM Plus for favorable estrogen metabolism, and GI supports such as IgG, Remove Complete, ParaKill, and CandiKill when microbial balance or gut inflammation is part of the picture.

Side-by-side lifestyle scenarios to help you choose. If you are a frequent flyer who forgets gels in hotel bathrooms and can't predict when you'll be able to give yourself an injection, pellets remove logistics from the equation and keep you even across time zones. If you love to tinker and want to self-adjust weekly based on gym performance, injections or transdermals may match your personality. If adhesives irritate your skin or you sweat off patches at work, pellets sidestep the problem. If you are training for a race with heavy lower-body work, plan insertions around your peak weeks. If finances are tight this season, consider starting with a lower-friction route and switching to pellets once your dose is predictable—there's more than one right path.

Common troubleshooting in human language. If hot flashes creep back two weeks before your reinsertion is due, your interval is a bit too long; shorten it next cycle. If sleep is deep but afternoon energy slumps, look at thyroid conversion, protein at breakfast, hydration, and magnesium timing before blaming pellets. If libido is strong but recovery is slow, evaluate training load and consider a growth-hormone supportive peptide cycle. If mood feels tight, check free testosterone and estradiol balance, stress rhythm, and SHBG. If a site feels tender beyond a week, check activity restrictions and talk to your provider to rule out irritation vs. infection.

A word on quality and trust. Pellets are only as good as the hands that place them and the pharmacy that compounds them. Work with experienced clinicians who place pellets regularly, monitor thoughtfully, and adjust conservatively. Ask how they calculate dose, how they time follow-ups, and how they manage the first two cycles. The goal is the smallest dose that restores function, not the biggest dose that creates a temporary "high." Precision is the prestige.

Long-term vision: what steady looks like over years. The real magic of pellets shows up over seasons. With a consistent signal, sleep consolidates, body composition trends leaner with training, bones see regular load and respond, brain fog lifts and stays gone, and the stress response becomes less hair-trigger. It's not a sprint; it's an architectural project—rebuilding capacity layer by layer so your later decades are not defined by managing decline but by enjoying competence, clarity, and connection.

Readiness checklist, conversational style. Ask yourself: Do I want fewer weekly health decisions? Does a minor procedure every few months fit my life? Am I willing to pair pellets with nutrition, training, sleep, and periodic labs? Do I prefer steadiness over day-to-day tweaking? If you're nodding along, pellets likely fit you. If you bristle at the idea of waiting until the next insertion to change dose, another route may serve you better now—with the option to switch later.

Questions people actually ask. Will I feel like "someone else"? The plan is designed to restore you to yourself, not turn you into a caricature. What if the dose is wrong? We adjust next cycle and use interval length as a fine-tuner; most people find their groove within one or two insertions. Does it hurt? It's quick, numbed, and feels more like pressure than pain; mild soreness fades in days. Can I remove a pellet if I don't like it? Pellets dissolve naturally; if a dose overshoots, the solution is to wait it out while adjusting timing next round. Can I swim or train? Yes—after the short initial restriction window your provider outlines. How soon will I notice changes? Sleep and evenness often shift within two weeks; body composition and bone density are longer arcs.

Final perspective. The point isn't the pellet. It's the life you build on top of a steady signal—deep sleep that shows up on schedule, mornings that begin on green, workouts that reward your effort, relationships with more patience and presence, and a physical body that feels like a good home again. Pellets are a tool. Used wisely, they make living your plan easier, not harder. The rest of this book will continue to show you how to stack the fundamentals—nutrition, training, gut health, stress rhythm, targeted supplements, and peptides—on top of hormone steadiness so you can age with intention and vigor.

Chapter 6

BHRT for Women: Rebalancing Estrogen, Progesterone & Testosterone Across Life Stages

The gentle truth most women never hear at a routine appointment is this: the way you feel right now is not "just your age." If you wake at three in the morning and stare at the ceiling, if your patience thins by late afternoon, if your waistline expands despite eating the way you always have, if names you know you know slip away mid-sentence, nothing about that means you're failing or falling apart. It means your biochemistry is trying to get your attention. Hormones are the body's master signals. They tell your brain how to sleep and focus, your metabolism how to burn and build, your muscles how to repair, your blood vessels how to relax, your bones how to remodel, your skin and vaginal tissues how to stay supple, and your desire how to wake up. When these signals fade or fall out of sync—first subtly in the late thirties, then more boldly in the forties and fifties—you don't become "less you." You become a woman whose operating system needs a tune-up.

Start with estrogen, because its reach is everywhere. Estradiol, the most active form, doesn't just affect hot flashes and periods; it is a brain, heart, bone, skin, and pelvic-tissue hormone. In the brain it stabilizes serotonin and dopamine, steadies temperature control, and keeps verbal memory crisp. In blood vessels it improves nitric-oxide signaling, which translates into better circulation and smoother blood pressure patterns when you're doing your part with food and movement. In bone it keeps turnover balanced so you build as much as you break down. In the skin and the entire genitourinary system it supports collagen, elasticity, moisture, and a healthy microbiome. When estradiol drifts low, sleep fragments, joints feel older than you are, urogenital tissues become dry and fragile, and a fog creeps into the edges of thought. You can white-knuckle your way through that for a while, but it steals energy you could spend on the life you actually want.

Progesterone is the nervous system's exhale. When you ovulate regularly, progesterone rises in the second half of the cycle and whispers calm to your brain, partnering with GABA—the body's internal anti-anxiety signal—to help you fall asleep and stay there. As ovulation becomes erratic in perimenopause, progesterone is often the first domino to wobble. The clues are familiar to millions of women: wired-and-tired evenings, tender breasts, heavier or more unpredictable bleeding, premenstrual irritability or anxiety, and that cruel two-to-three-a.m. wake-up. Bioidentical micronized progesterone at bedtime often feels like the "ahhh" your system has been missing: sleep deepens, ruminating thoughts quiet, and the luteal half of the month becomes livable again. If you use systemic estrogen and you still have a uterus, progesterone does another job too—protecting the endometrium and keeping therapy safe by design.

Then there's testosterone. Yes, women make it—less than men, but not less important. When female-physiologic testosterone is too low, drive—physical and mental—slumps. Workouts feel flat no matter how disciplined you are. Midsection weight is suddenly stubborn. Sexual desire needs scheduling instead of arriving unannounced. Orgasm may be slower or less intense. Restoring a woman's testosterone to a healthy female range has a very specific feel: mornings start with forward momentum instead of a fight, exercise starts paying you back, waistlines trim with the same effort that used to maintain, and desire returns as a spark rather than a chore. Optimized alongside estradiol and progesterone, testosterone often steadies mood and makes the whole stress response less hair-trigger.

Two more hormones deserve the front row because they shape how the above feel in real life: thyroid and DHEA. Thyroid sets your metabolic tempo. If you can't convert T4 to the active T3 well—because of inflammation, nutrient gaps, chronic stress, or gut issues—everything feels like swimming upstream. Cold hands and feet, constipation, hair shedding, dry skin, slow thinking, flat mood, and weight that refuses to budge are the greatest hits. DHEA is quieter but just as meaningful; it's a resilience hormone that also contributes to libido and immune balance. When DHEA is low, stress hits harder and you recover slower from illness or big life pushes. None of these systems live in isolation. Restore one, and you often make the others easier to optimize. Ignore one, and you can end up pushing the gas with one foot and the brake with the other.

The way these hormones change isn't the same for every woman, but there are patterns. Late thirties into early forties is a tricky zone because cycles can look perfectly regular on a calendar while luteal progesterone is already running low. The lived experience is sleep disruption the week before your period, heavier flow, new PMS patterns, and a kind of invisible edge that wasn't there before. The solution starts with timing-appropriate labs to confirm ovulation and luteal progesterone, but you don't have to wait for perfect paperwork to support your system. A protein-forward, low-inflammatory diet, two to three days a week of progressive strength training, morning light exposure, and magnesium at night create the terrain where hormones behave better. If luteal progesterone is indeed low, nighttime bioidentical progesterone can transform those last ten days of the cycle from "survive" to "fine."

Perimenopause—the mid-forties through early fifties for many—is a physiology rollercoaster. Estradiol can soar and crash; progesterone is often simply not there; and androgens trend downward, which you feel as sluggishness in the gym and stubborn weight in the mirror. Thyroid conversion may wobble under the strain of poor sleep and higher stress. The working strategy here is "stabilize and soothe." Nighttime progesterone to restore sleep and calm the nervous system. If hot flashes, brain fog, joint pain, or mood volatility are chewing through your days, systemic estradiol support with a non-oral route can steady the floor without running through your liver first. Pay attention to insulin and the gut—spiky blood sugar and a cranky microbiome amplify weight gain and mood swings—so keep protein high, fiber meaningful, and ultra-processed foods rare. This is also where peptides and targeted nutraceuticals can buy you momentum while lifestyle changes take root, because when sleep improves everything else gets easier.

Menopause—twelve months without a period—is not the end of the story; it's the start of a new, stable baseline. Without ovarian estradiol, thermoregulation, sleep, bone turnover, and urogenital tissues need explicit support if you want to protect your healthspan rather than just your lifespan. Many women do best on non-oral estradiol for systemic benefits, paired with progesterone at night (if they have a uterus) and a female-physiologic dose of testosterone for muscle, mood, and desire. Layer on strength and power training—your bones listen to load—and make sure protein intake is not the afterthought it was in your twenties. One and a half to two grams of protein per kilogram of body weight per day is a helpful target for active women reclaiming muscle and metabolic health. If you're rebuilding after surgical menopause or treatment-induced ovarian shutdown, think "sooner" for support; the body didn't have time to adapt, so you give it what it lost and build nervous-system steadiness quickly with structure, light timing, magnesium, and gentle breath work.

If you have a history of PCOS, you don't just "grow out of it." The insulin-androgen axis you met in your teens follows you into midlife. The midlife update is that cycles can become unpredictable for two reasons at once—perimenopausal hormone chaos on top of insulin resistance. The answer is unglamorous and effective: insulin sensitivity first. Build meals around protein, vegetables, and healthy fats; lift weights; walk daily; sleep like it matters. Omega-3s and magnesium take the edge off inflammation and help both insulin and mood behave. Nighttime progesterone can still be a gift even with a PCOS background because it's not only about the uterus; it's about the brain's ability to downshift and sleep. If baseline testosterone is already robust, you focus on estradiol-progesterone balance and metabolism before even considering androgens.

None of this works well if you test like a box-checker. Start with symptoms and goals, then let labs clarify. A smart baseline looks at estradiol with a sensitive assay, progesterone timed mid-luteal if you're cycling, total and free testosterone plus SHBG for bioavailability, DHEA-S for your stress backbone, and a full thyroid panel—not just TSH but free T4, free T3, sometimes reverse T3, and antibodies when it fits the picture. Add fasting insulin and glucose, A1C, a lipid panel with particle information when it's available, hs-CRP for inflammation, ferritin for iron stores, vitamin D for immune and bone sanity, and B12/folate to assess energy and methylation. Don't forget cortisol as a pattern across the day, because the curve is the message—high-all-day feels anxious and snack-seeking, low-all-day feels flat and salt-craving, and both make sex hormones feel worse. When you interpret, be suspicious of the word "normal." Normal ranges are population averages, and the population is not thriving. What matters is whether the numbers match how you sleep, think, recover, and perform. Your lived pattern is the endpoint.

Delivery route matters because real life matters. For most women, longer-acting pellets are the preferred route—especially for testosterone and, when appropriate, estradiol—because they provide steady, physiologic levels for months, remove daily decision fatigue, and smooth out peaks and troughs; the trade-offs are a brief in-office procedure, slower mid-cycle dose adjustments, and rare site irritation. Non-oral estradiol delivered by patches or gels also supports steady levels and avoids first-pass liver effects; the flipside is potential skin sensitivity, adhesive issues, and the need to remember daily or twice-weekly application. Oral estradiol remains a thoughtful option; it is simple and often affordable, yet it carries a different risk–benefit profile for some and does not bypass first-pass metabolism. Local vaginal estradiol is a tiny-dose, big-benefit addition for tissue comfort, pH balance, and sexual ease, helpful whether or not you choose systemic therapy, though it does not replace whole-body support. Progesterone is most often bioidentical and taken orally at bedtime because it partners well with sleep and protects the uterine lining when that is relevant; possible downsides include next-day grogginess or dizziness, and while vaginal formulations can be effective, they are usually messier. Testosterone can be delivered as low-dose creams or gels that are adjustable and noninvasive but require daily use and care to avoid transfer, as micro-dose injections that are precise yet can create small peaks, as troches or buccal forms that are easy but variably absorbed, or as longer-acting pellets—our preferred choice—for consistency and convenience. The goal is not more; the goal is yours—the dose that restores function without drifting into side effects like oily skin, acne, unwanted hair growth, or voice change. If those appear, we turn the dose down and the effects fade. You do not abandon a helpful hormone because a dial needed a nudge.

Peptides are not a replacement for hormones; they are a way to make your plan work better by improving sleep depth, recovery, tissue repair, mitochondrial output, and even central arousal. If your nights are fragmented, a short course of CJC-1295 with Ipamorelin—or a gentler nudge with Sermorelin—can deepen slow-wave sleep and shorten the distance between "lights out" and real rest. The downstream benefits are everywhere—better insulin sensitivity, steadier mood, and easier thyroid conversion the next day. If long-standing aches are the reason you're avoiding the gym, BPC-157 supports tendon, ligament, muscle, and gut healing, while KPV adds local anti-inflammatory help for the gut and skin; a combination that includes TB-based repair signals can accelerate the feeling that your body will hold up to the training you know you need. Body-composition needles can be nudged with Tesamorelin when visceral fat is the enemy, with MOTS-C plus AICAR when you want mitochondrial efficiency so walks turn into actual fat-burning and workouts stop feeling like chores, and with AOD9604 when you want fat-metabolism support without altering growth hormone directly. For focus and mood during hormonal transitions, curated brain stacks—NAD+ with BDNF and Alpha-GPC or broader blends that add Selank, Semax, oxytocin, huperzine, and dihexa under professional guidance—can clear the fog enough that your other upgrades stick. PT-141 is especially meaningful for women whose desire lags despite adequate estradiol and testosterone, because it works centrally on arousal rather than relying on the plumbing alone. And if you want the outside to reflect the inside, GHK-Cu supports collagen and hair fullness, and blends that combine it with healing signals can help skin recover while you do the internal work with hormones, protein, and micronutrients.

Nutraceuticals are the building materials and enzyme helpers that let hormone signals "land." Comprehensive female-focused formulas such as Women's Complete and Women's Vitality are designed to cover the essentials women commonly lack—bioavailable minerals for thyroid and metabolic enzymes; the full B-family in methylated forms for energy, neurotransmitter balance, and methylation; antioxidant support to buffer oxidative stress; and targeted botanicals chosen for stress resilience, healthy inflammatory balance, and hormone metabolism. Think of these as daily scaffolding that makes your biology easier to live in. Estrogen metabolism also benefits from diindolylmethane (DIM) nudging pathways in favorable directions; vitamins A, D3, and K2 support bone mineralization, vascular integrity, immune balance, and receptor function so the message gets through; and omega-3s cool the inflammatory noise that scrambles signals while supporting brain and joint comfort. If energy and mood are wobbly, a methylated B-complex smooths the weekly grind. Magnesium at night deepens rest, reduces nighttime muscle tension, and steadies the stress response. For women whose thyroid symptoms become obvious once estradiol and progesterone are steadier, a formula that supplies iodine (when appropriate), selenium, zinc, and iron sufficiency helps T4 turn into the T3 you actually feel. And because the gut-immune axis either amplifies or sabotages hormone work, it needs its own attention: immunoglobulin G formulas bind and escort inflammatory fragments; comprehensive resets help tame microbial overgrowth; targeted tools address parasites or candida when they show up; and mucosal repair blends help rebuild the barrier so you absorb what you swallow and the estrogen–gut conversation (the "estrobolome") stays friendly rather than feeding symptoms.

None of this lives in a vacuum. Sleep is hormone therapy. Seven to nine hours of consolidated sleep is when progesterone's calm and estradiol's brain repair become lived experience rather than theory. Build a simple, stubborn routine: morning light within an hour of waking to anchor your circadian clock; an eight-hour caffeine cutoff before bedtime; protein and magnesium at dinner to keep blood sugar smooth and muscles relaxed; dim the house; keep the bedroom cool, dark, and quiet; and banish glowing rectangles from the pillows. If perimenopause is sabotaging this effort, use nocturnal progesterone, consider the right dose and route of estradiol, and add a short sleep-supportive peptide cycle while foundations take hold. Chronic stress is a hormone story too; it steals from progesterone's calm and flattens estradiol signaling. Create a rhythm you'll actually do: a protein-first breakfast, a couple of daylight walks, resistance training earlier in the day, a brief evening stroll outside to mark "work is over," a breath practice you enjoy instead of endure, and magnesium-anchored wind-down. Calm daytime formulas help when your calendar runs hot, and adrenal-rebuilding blends restore a stronger morning peak after a burnout chapter. Strength training is not optional if you care about female hormones. Muscle is your glucose storage, your hormone-sensitivity organ, and your longevity insurance. Two to three resistance sessions per week—compound lifts, progressive overload—plus daily walking and a sprinkle of power bring back a body that listens. If joints complain, let connective-tissue peptides support repair so you don't stall. When hormones are optimized, training begins to pay you back again—faster recovery, steadier effort, better composition changes at the same calorie intake.

Eat like someone rebuilding tissue. A useful target for active women reclaiming strength is roughly 1.6 to 2.0 grams of protein per kilogram of body weight per day, anchored evenly across meals. Build plates around high-quality protein, add colorful plants and fiber for estrogen metabolism and gut health, and include healthy fats—olive oil, avocado, egg yolks, nuts—for membranes and the steroid hormone backbone. Watch how cravings quiet as insulin sensitivity returns. Grain-heavy, ultra-processed patterns drive the opposite: blood-sugar swings, inflammation, cravings that look like "lack of discipline" but are really chemistry. This isn't a moral issue; it's physics. Put the right materials on the table and your physiology becomes easier to live in. Don't, and you'll keep fighting yourself.

It helps to picture how this plays out in real lives. A forty-five-year-old project manager and runner drifts awake at three a.m. every night, premenstrual anxiety turns the second half of the month into an ordeal, and a new ring of belly fat doesn't budge. Tests show low luteal progesterone, fluctuating estradiol, very low free testosterone, borderline ferritin, and insulin creeping higher. Nighttime micronized progesterone restores deep sleep within two weeks. A low-dose transdermal estradiol calms the thermoregulation swings. A physiologic female dose of testosterone cream brings back gym traction. A methylated B-complex, vitamins A/D/K2, omega-3s, and magnesium fill in the gaps. Protein climbs to 120 grams per day and strength training happens twice a week. A short cycle of growth-hormone secretagogues deepens slow-wave sleep. Eight weeks later she wakes before her alarm and moves through days without white-knuckling.

A fifty-three-year-old teacher in natural menopause shows up with hot flashes, brain fog, vaginal dryness and pain with intercourse, and weight gain despite daily walks. Estradiol and progesterone are low, free testosterone is low, TSH looks "fine" but free T3 is also low, vitamin D is deficient, and inflammation markers are up. A non-oral estradiol route steadies the floor. Nighttime progesterone helps her sleep and protects her uterus. A tiny female dose of testosterone returns desire and exercise payoffs. A small T3 addition with thyroid-supportive nutrients warms her hands and clears her head. Vitamins A/D/K2, omega-3s, and magnesium round out the basics. Pelvic-floor rehab plus local vaginal estradiol and, if desired, platelet-rich plasma injections guided by an experienced clinician restore tissue comfort and sexual ease. Three months later hot flashes are rare and brief, intercourse is comfortable, and weight begins to normalize as sleep turns into a superpower again.

A thirty-nine-year-old with a PCOS history enters perimenopause and thinks she's back in high school—irregular cycles, acne, sugar cravings, and low desire. Insulin is elevated, SHBG is low, free testosterone is low-normal, estradiol is variable. The plan is metabolic first: protein and fiber at every meal, daily walking, and strength training. Omega-3s and magnesium dampen inflammation and help cravings lose their hold. Nighttime progesterone repairs sleep and premenstrual mood. Estradiol support is cautious and physiologic when symptoms demand it. Testosterone waits. BPC-157 and KPV calm a reactive gut and inflammatory skin flares. In three months, cycles are more predictable, cravings recede, skin settles, and desire starts to show up on its own.

Along the way you'll have questions, and the answers are almost always kinder than the internet suggests. Tender breasts after starting estrogen often mean tissues are waking up, not that you're in danger. Keep the dose physiologic, support metabolism with DIM, confirm progesterone at night, and re-assess at six to eight weeks instead of two. If testosterone gives you your drive back but makes your skin a bit oilier, you're probably near the top of your sweet spot. Ease the dose down; it's fixable. If your labs say "normal" and you feel textbook hypothyroid, look past TSH to free T3, ferritin, selenium, zinc, and inflammation, then support conversion and rest. If stubborn belly fat is the headline, look at insulin, sleep, cortisol rhythm, and thyroid conversion before you blame estrogen. If orgasm is elusive even when libido is okay, evaluate pelvic-floor tone and vaginal tissue health, consider local estradiol even on systemic therapy, and remember that central arousal support can be layered when needed. If you've had a hysterectomy but kept your ovaries, progesterone can still be your friend because it's as much a brain and sleep hormone as it is a uterine one.

If this sounds like work, that's because it is—but it's the good kind, the kind that pays compound interest. Test like a detective, not a box-checker. Restore signals at physiologic levels using routes you can sustain. Keep thyroid, DHEA, insulin, and cortisol in the room because they decide how the others feel. Build behaviors that actually fit your life: a stubborn sleep routine, strength training you'll honor, protein-forward meals that satisfy, walks that anchor your days, sunlight that tells your clock what time it is. Support with nutraceuticals that make biology easier and with peptides that protect momentum when life is chaotic. Monitor and adjust with your lived experience as the North Star—sleep, mood, energy, body composition, cognition, and desire—then let labs confirm the pattern you already feel.

You don't need perfect biology to live well. You need biology that listens. Female hormone optimization is about giving your body the right messages in the right amounts at the right times so it can hear you again. The payoff isn't just fewer hot flashes or less belly fat or a less combative calendar; it's the return of a self you recognize: clear-minded, strong, affectionate, patient, and creative. That woman is not gone. She was waiting for a physiology that supports her. This is how you build it, at any age.

Chapter 7

BHRT for Men: Strength, Clarity, and Metabolism at Every Age

If you're a man who's losing your edge—dragging through the afternoon, snapping at the people you love, skipping the gym because your joints ache and your drive is gone—you're not "failing at discipline." You're hearing a biological signal. The modern story men are told is that this feeling is inevitable: you hit your forties or fifties, gain a gut, trade muscle for stiffness, and make peace with a shrinking life. That story is convenient for industries that sell quick fixes for symptoms, but it's not how the body has to age. When you understand what hormones actually do—and restore them to the ranges your body recognizes—energy returns, composition shifts, and confidence stops being something you have to psych yourself into.

Testosterone sits at the center of that change, but the full picture is wider. In a healthy male physiology, testosterone is the voice that tells muscle to grow, the brain to focus, the mitochondria to produce energy, and the libido to wake up. When levels fall, the symptoms are rarely subtle: morning erections fade, strength gains stall, work requires more caffeine than it used to, patience thins, and body fat migrates to the midsection no matter how much cardio you add. Yet it's not just testosterone that matters. Men need small but well-timed amounts of estradiol—made from testosterone via aromatase—to keep joints lubricated, the brain sharp, and the cardiovascular system responsive. When estradiol falls too low from aggressive suppression, men feel brittle: joint aches, flat mood, and a libido that looks normal on paper but doesn't show up in real life. Dihydrotestosterone (DHT) matters, too. It's more potent at the androgen receptor and contributes to drive and genital sensitivity; the goal isn't zero DHT but a balanced range with close attention to prostate health. Layer in thyroid to set metabolic tempo, DHEA for resilience and immune tone, insulin for fuel partitioning, and cortisol for stress rhythm—and you have the network that determines whether your body cooperates or resists you.

Most men start this journey because of how they feel, not because of a number. Still, smart testing gives you the map you need to navigate. A useful baseline includes total and free testosterone with SHBG so you know what's actually available to tissues; estradiol by a sensitive assay; DHT; LH and FSH to understand testicular signaling; prolactin when libido is low or gynecomastia has appeared; a complete thyroid panel (TSH, free T4, free T3, and sometimes reverse T3 and antibodies); fasting insulin and glucose with A1C to frame metabolism; a lipid panel with particle information when available; hs-CRP for inflammation; ferritin and CBC for iron/hematocrit; vitamin D and B12/folate for energy and immune support; and a PSA with digital exam to set a prostate baseline. If fertility is a priority, include semen analysis before any therapy. Numbers don't get the final vote—your lived experience does—but good labs let you personalize care and monitor safety with confidence.

The goal of bioidentical hormone replacement therapy (BHRT) in men is not to chase a "bodybuilder" range or mask a lifestyle that's working against you. It's to restore a physiologic signal you can live on. Delivery route is about the life you have, not someone else's preference. Injections work exceptionally well when dosed with a micro-schedule—smaller amounts two to three times per week to keep peaks and troughs flat. Weekly or bi-weekly boluses create a rollercoaster: two days high, three days low, a day when you think therapy "stopped working," and then the cycle repeats. Transdermal creams and gels make small day-to-day adjustments easy but require consistent application and drying time; absorption varies with skin thickness, sweat, and shower timing. Troches deliver quick, flexible dosing but may create intra-day rises and falls some men can feel. Pellets trade day-to-day dosing for months of even release, which is ideal for men who travel constantly or dislike needles; as we covered previously, dose and interval are tuned across the first one to two cycles and then the plan tends to run on rails. Oral testosterone options exist but are less commonly used long-term because of variability or hepatic considerations in some formulations. None of these is "right" for everyone. The right route is the one you will use consistently and happily.

Estradiol in men deserves a special, clear conversation because it's often misunderstood. Men do best when estradiol lands in a healthy, physiologic range—high enough to support brain, bone, joint, and sexual health; not so high that it drives water retention or breast tissue tenderness. The reflex to block aromatase with medication every time estradiol rises on a lab report often creates more problems than it solves. Before reaching for a blocker, look at dose and delivery (is your testosterone peaking too high between shots?), body fat (visceral adipose is an aromatase factory), alcohol intake (which raises aromatase), sleep and stress (which alter conversion), and nutrition (which shapes insulin and inflammation). Many men normalize estradiol by flattening their testosterone curve with micro-dosing, trimming visceral fat with protein-forward eating and strength training, and reducing alcohol—all without sacrificing the benefits of aromatization. There are cases where medication is indicated, but it should be a thoughtful, minimal tool rather than a default.

Safety is not a headline; it's a pattern you build into care. Hematocrit can rise on testosterone because androgens stimulate red blood cell production; you monitor it and adjust dose/intervals or donate if needed. If you snore heavily or wake unrefreshed, evaluate sleep apnea because untreated apnea amplifies blood pressure and hematocrit issues. Prostate health requires a baseline and periodic PSA with clinical context; the data support that restoring physiologic testosterone does not "feed" prostate cancer, but men with a history of cancer need coordinated care with their urologist. Lipids, blood pressure, and insulin sensitivity often improve with muscle gain and fat loss on BHRT, but they still deserve attention. Mood and behavioral shifts—irritability, impulsivity—usually mean the dose is too high for you or the curve is too peaky; flattening the schedule or reducing the dose restores steadiness.

The red line is simple: the smallest dose that restores function, paired with the behaviors that make the dose work for you instead of against you.

Fertility requires its own path because exogenous testosterone suppresses sperm production. If you want to conceive in the near-to-medium term, you typically avoid direct testosterone and instead support your own production with agents like hCG or enclomiphene, sometimes with FSH under specialist care. If you're already on testosterone and want to restore fertility, a structured plan with those same tools can wake the axis back up. None of this is guesswork; you work from semen parameters and labs rather than hope and frustration.

Peptides are the precision tools that protect your momentum while hormones and habits do the heavy lifting. If you need deeper sleep and faster recovery, growth-hormone secretagogues like CJC-1295 with Ipamorelin—or a gentler Sermorelin—can deepen slow-wave sleep, reduce next-day soreness, and make training feel rewarding again. If your joints and tendons are the bottleneck, BPC-157 supports tissue repair from the inside out, TB-500 helps reduce inflammation around overused structures, and a BPC-157/TB blend is a pragmatic recovery stack during high-volume training phases. If your goal is to target visceral fat without sacrificing lean mass, Tesamorelin is particularly helpful; paired with protein-forward nutrition and resistance training, men often notice waist measurements shifting before the scale moves. For global metabolic and endurance benefits, the mitochondrial duo MOTS-C + AICAR nudges cells to burn fuel more efficiently so long runs and hill repeats stop feeling like punishment. AOD9604 adds a fat-metabolism nudge that doesn't alter growth hormone directly. For sexual function, PT-141 acts centrally on arousal pathways and can be a meaningful adjunct when desire lags despite a healthy testosterone/estradiol balance; Melanotan II has similar melanocortin activity with the aesthetic side effect of tanning. For cognition and drive, blends that combine NAD+ with BDNF support and Alpha-GPC sharpen mental energy and task initiation; comprehensive stacks like Brain Ultra 7 (which may include Selank, Semax, oxytocin, alpha-GPC, huperzine, BDNF support, and dihexa) can raise the ceiling on focus and stress resilience during high-demand seasons. For skin and hair, GHK-Cu encourages collagen and scalp vitality; a "Glow"-style blend that layers GHK-Cu with healing peptides can help the outside reflect the inside as metabolism and training come back online.

Nutraceuticals make hormone signals easier to use because they supply the cofactors your enzymes need and the buffers your tissues rely on. A daily men's foundation—think comprehensive "Men's Complete" and a performance-leaning "Men's Vitality"—covers gaps in magnesium, zinc, selenium, and trace minerals; delivers methylated B vitamins for energy, methylation, and neurotransmitter balance; and adds supportive antioxidants and botanicals for healthy inflammation control and stress handling. Vitamin D3 with K2 and vitamin A in a balanced formula (ADK10 or ADK5) supports bone mineralization, vascular integrity, immune tone, and receptor signaling so testosterone's message lands at the cell. Omega-3s (Super Omega 3D) cool inflammatory noise, protect joints, and support cardiovascular and brain health—especially important when you're training hard again. Magnesium

("Mag Complete") deepens sleep, eases post-workout muscle tone, and steadies the stress response. If estrogen metabolism needs nudging because estradiol is high relative to how you feel, a diindolylmethane complex (DIM Plus) can help shift pathways without crashing levels. Thyroid cofactors matter more than most men expect; a thoughtful blend ("Thyroid Complete") that includes iodine when appropriate, selenium, zinc, and iron sufficiency allows T4-to-T3 conversion to do its job. DHEA, used judiciously and titrated by labs and symptoms, can restore a sense of resilience and sexual interest in men who run low.

Gut health is often the missing amplifier. An inflamed gut blunts nutrient absorption, elevates cortisol, and recycles estrogens in ways that make you feel puffy and irritable. If your digestion is noisy—bloating, irregular stools, reflux, fatigue after meals—address that first. Immunoglobulin G (IgG) formulas help bind and escort inflammatory fragments out of the gut; a structured reset ("Remove Complete") calms microbial overgrowth; targeted tools like "ParaKill" for parasites and "CandiKill" for yeast address specific patterns when indicated; and mucosal repair blends ("GI Complete") help rebuild the barrier so the food you prioritize actually nourishes you. Men are famous for ignoring early gut signals; in BHRT, ignoring them is like trying to drive with the parking brake on.

Sleep and stress are the multipliers of everything else. Seven to nine hours of consolidated sleep turns testosterone into lived experience—morning drive, stable mood, spontaneous erections, stronger lifts, better glucose control. Build a predictable rhythm: morning light within an hour of waking, resistance training earlier in the day, a caffeine cutoff eight hours before bed, protein and magnesium at dinner, and an electronics-free last hour in a dark, cool room. If stress is running hot, daytime composure support ("Calm Day") keeps your brain from redlining; when burnout has flattened your morning energy, adrenal support ("AdrenaMax" or "Adrenal Restore") helps rebuild a healthy cortisol peak so you can wake without a chemical shove. If sleep is the last domino, a simple "Sleep Time" formula can nudge you into deeper stages while foundation work takes hold. None of these replace habits; they make the habits stick.

Training is where you turn chemistry into capability. Muscle is not a vanity metric; it's your glucose sink, your joint stabilizer, and your longevity engine. Two to three days per week of progressive resistance training, a daily walking target, and a sprinkle of power work (sprints, loaded carries, jumps you can land safely) rebuild the body that carries your life. With hormones restored, recovery accelerates and aches shrink; with peptides and omega-3s in the background, connective tissue holds up. Protein needs rise when you train and when you're trying to reverse years of under-recovery; a practical target for many men is ~1.6–2.2 g/kg/day, distributed across meals. This isn't punishment; it's permission to rebuild.

To see how this plays out, picture three men you might recognize. The first is a 38-year-old founder who has been living on caffeine and adrenaline for a decade. He's still lean, but he's exhausted by 3 p.m., irritable at home, and watching his lifts slide. Labs show total testosterone in the low-normal range, free testosterone low because SHBG is high, estradiol low-normal, a flat diurnal cortisol curve, and ferritin on the low side from a minimalist diet. He moves to micro-dosed injections twice weekly, adds nighttime magnesium and a sleep discipline, and uses CJC-1295 with Ipamorelin for six weeks to deepen slow-wave sleep. Men's Complete and Men's Vitality fill mineral and B-vitamin gaps; ADK10 and Super Omega 3D create an anti-inflammatory backdrop; Calm Day tames the late-day spikes. Four weeks later, he's less reactive, and his wife says she "has her husband back."

The second is a 56-year-old executive who used to be an athlete. He's on blood pressure and lipid medications, wakes to urinate twice nightly, and has stopped initiating sex because his confidence evaporated. Total testosterone is 320 ng/dL with free in the basement, estradiol is high relative to how he feels, insulin is elevated, A1C is creeping, hematocrit is high-normal, and sleep apnea is probable. He starts with a sleep study and CPAP while shifting to a protein-forward diet and daily walks. Testosterone is begun with a transdermal route while habits lock; once consistent, he transitions to micro-dosed injections. Estradiol normalizes as visceral fat falls and the curve flattens; DIM Plus supports metabolism without medicating aromatase. BPC-157/TB stack lets him lift again without flaring tendons. ADK10, Super Omega 3D, and Mag Complete round out the essentials; Thyroid Complete is added once labs show subpar T3 conversion. Six months later, his belt is two holes tighter, blood pressure and lipids are improving with less medication, and morning erections are back.

The third is a 44-year-old teacher who wants a second child. He has all the symptoms of low T but doesn't want to risk fertility. Instead of exogenous testosterone, he starts enclomiphene with hCG, fixes sleep and nutrition, and trains consistently. PT-141 helps confidence and central arousal while the axis recovers. Within a few months, semen parameters improve, his mood steadies, and he says that for the first time in years his "get-up-and-go got up and went."

Along the way, questions come up that have simple, respectful answers. "Will testosterone make me aggressive?" Not at physiologic doses that fit your life and labs; feeling irritable usually means your curve is peaky or your dose is too high for you. "Will I need this forever?" You will need a plan for as long as you want the benefits. For some men that's BHRT; for others, it's lifestyle plus supportive agents while they recover endogenous production. "Isn't estrogen bad for men?" No—men with estradiol that's too low feel brittle and underperform. The goal is balance, not suppression. "What about the prostate?" You set a baseline, monitor, and place the numbers in clinical context. Healthy, steady-state testosterone paired with muscle gain, fat loss, and better sleep tends to move risk in the right direction. "What about heart risk?" Body composition, insulin sensitivity, blood pressure, and lipids generally improve when you restore hormones and live like it matters. Monitoring isn't optional, but fear doesn't have to be your plan.

When you pull back, a through-line appears. You test like a detective, restore signals at physiologic levels, choose a route that fits your day, and build behaviors that make chemistry tangible: protein-forward meals, ironed-in sleep, progressive strength, walks that anchor your nervous system, and sunlight to set your clock. You protect momentum with peptides when you need a bridge. You support the machinery with targeted nutraceuticals. You watch the markers that matter—sleep, mood, libido, strength, waist circumference, fasting glucose, hematocrit, blood pressure, PSA—and you adjust before problems grow teeth. None of this turns you into someone else. It returns you to yourself: stronger, steadier, clearer, kinder, and more present in the life you've worked hard to build.

Aging is inevitable; decline is negotiable. For men, the negotiation gets easier when hormones, habits, and tools are aligned. This isn't a game of hacks or shortcuts. It's a decision to live with a full signal—day after day, season after season—so your biology works with you instead of against you. Do that consistently and the changes stop being "results." They become your new baseline.

Chapter 8

Peptides: The Future of Regenerative Medicine

If you're doing everything "right"—eating better, lifting weights, dialing in sleep—and still feel like your body isn't cashing the check, you're not imagining it. There is a gap between effort and outcome for many people in midlife. The body is willing, but the signals that direct repair, fat loss, focus, and recovery are faint. That's the problem peptides are designed to solve. They are not a shortcut around fundamentals; they're the precision tools that make the fundamentals work the way they're supposed to. When you restore hormonal signals with BHRT and then layer in the right peptides, you're not forcing biology—you're reminding it. The result is a body that heals faster, trains harder, sleeps deeper, burns cleaner, and thinks clearer.

A peptide is a short chain of amino acids—shorter than a protein—that your body already understands. Because peptides mimic or amplify your own signaling molecules, they nudge biology rather than bulldoze it. That's the key difference from many pharmaceuticals designed to override pathways. With a well-chosen peptide, you're tapping a dormant circuit: "heal this tendon," "release a pulse of growth hormone at night," "switch on mitochondrial fat-burning," "tighten collagen," "turn down gut inflammation," or "wake up central arousal." This is why people often describe peptides as "subtle but steady." You don't feel whiplash. You feel traction.

Think of peptide families as specialized crews. Healing peptides direct tissue repair and reduce inflammation—this is where BPC-157, TB-500 (a fragment of thymosin beta-4), and blends that combine them shine. Metabolic and mitochondrial peptides improve how you produce and use energy—MOTS-C, AICAR, and AOD9604 live here, along with tesamorelin, which targets visceral fat while preserving lean mass. Growth-hormone secretagogues such as CJC-1295 paired with Ipamorelin (or a gentler Sermorelin) cue your own pituitary to release pulses of growth hormone—especially at night—so sleep, recovery, and body composition improve together. Neurocognitive and mood-supportive peptides—Selank, Semax, NAD+ / BDNF / Alpha-GPC blends, and comprehensive nootropic stacks—restore calm focus under pressure. Central arousal peptides (PT-141, Melanotan II) help when hormones are "fine on paper" but desire is missing. Aesthetic peptides like GHK-Cu improve skin and hair by signaling collagen synthesis and follicle vitality.

What makes peptides different is their "do one thing well" design. BPC-157, for example, is famous among athletes and everyday movers because it supports angiogenesis (new blood vessels in healing tissue), orchestrates collagen organization, and damps inflammatory cascades that keep tendons and fascia angry. People notice fewer "zingy" pains, better tolerance for progressive loading, and the confidence to return to the movements that build muscle and protect joints. TB-500 complements that by improving cell migration and speeding tissue remodeling—especially useful in overuse patterns that never quite finish healing. Used together around a rehab plan, they turn "it's always irritated" into "I can load it again."

Metabolism has its own language, and mitochondrial peptides translate it. MOTS-C upregulates pathways that make your cells more metabolically flexible—better at burning fat when you ask them to, better at sparing glucose for the brain when you need clarity. AICAR acts like a cellular "low fuel" signal (AMPK activation), nudging the body to increase glucose uptake and fatty-acid oxidation. Pair these with strength training and a protein-forward diet and hills feel shorter, zone-2 work stops being a grind, and the same number on a scale hides a very different waist measurement. For stubborn visceral fat, tesamorelin is a targeted lever that preserves lean mass while shrinking the riskier fat around organs. For a gentler nudge without altering growth hormone directly, AOD9604 focuses on fat metabolism with an excellent tolerance profile.

Sleep and recovery are where many wellness plans fail—not because people don't care, but because their nervous systems have forgotten how to downshift. Growth-hormone secretagogues are the quiet fix. CJC-1295 paired with Ipamorelin sends a "now" message to your pituitary to release natural pulses of growth hormone, especially at night. People don't describe a jolt; they describe falling asleep faster, sleeping deeper, waking with less soreness, and getting more out of the same training. That's the point: you're amplifying your own physiology, not replacing it. Sermorelin is a gentler option some prefer when they want a lower-octane nudge with similar sleep benefits.

Brain fog isn't a character flaw—it's chemistry. Neurocognitive peptides address it from multiple angles. Selank and Semax are anxiolytic, pro-cognitive signals many experience as "calm focus": less background static, more executive function under stress. NAD+ combinations with BDNF support and Alpha-GPC provide the energy and plasticity side—more mitochondrial output for the neurons you already have and better growth signals for synapses to strengthen. Thoughtfully curated stacks that layer those elements (and, where appropriate, oxytocin, huperzine, and dihexa) help people feel like their brains are "online" again when life is demanding.

Sexual health is one of the most honest readouts of whole-system vitality. You can't fake libido for long; your brain decides. PT-141 acts centrally on melanocortin receptors to support arousal in both men and women. Unlike peripheral agents that rely on blood-flow mechanics alone, PT-141 addresses desire, which is why it can help when hormones are "fine on paper" but life has turned your brain's interest down. Melanotan II has similar central activity with a cosmetic tan as a side effect, which some people appreciate and others avoid.

Skin and hair telegraph health. GHK-Cu, a naturally occurring copper peptide, binds to receptors in the skin to promote collagen synthesis, wound healing, and hair follicle vitality. People notice "paper" texture soften, fine lines blur, and thinning patches look fuller. When you're rebuilding your body from the inside with protein, strength training, and steady hormones, it's satisfying to see the outside keep pace.

Peptides are not magic. They are leverage. They work best when you give them the basics to work with: protein sufficiency so repair has bricks and mortar, resistance training so the body is told what structure to build, sleep rhythms so pulses happen at the right time, and foundational micronutrients so enzymes can do their jobs. When those are present, the right peptide turns the dial in your favor faster than lifestyle alone. Strategically, peptides are adjuncts to BHRT, not substitutes. Hormones set the operating system; peptides write targeted patches that fix bottlenecks in performance and recovery.

Here's how to match goals to peptides without turning your life into a chemistry hobby. If you're constantly sore or dealing with repeat injuries, start with healing signals: BPC-157 for connective tissue and gut, and TB-based support if you've had troublesome tendons or fascia. If your main frustration is that cardio feels harder than it should and the scale ignores your effort, consider MOTS-C + AICAR for mitochondrial efficiency and AOD9604 for gentle fat nudging; layer tesamorelin if visceral fat is the issue. If sleep is the bottleneck, choose CJC-1295 + Ipamorelin or Sermorelin during high-stress seasons to restore deep sleep and faster recovery. If focus and mood are wobbling, lean on NAD+ / BDNF / Alpha-GPC or add Selank/Semax under guidance. If desire is missing even when hormones look good, PT-141 can reconnect the brain to the body. If skin quality and hair fullness trail your internal progress, add GHK-Cu and consider blends that include a healing signal for better dermal remodeling.

Stacking and cycling matter because receptors like rhythm and you like results. Most peptides are used in defined windows—typically six to twelve weeks for a goal, then time off. Some, like BPC-157, are pulsed around a training cycle or injury period. Others, like GHK-Cu for skin, can become part of a longer routine with periodic breaks. Growth-hormone secretagogues deliver the most in the first few months as sleep normalizes and tissue turnover improves; many people return to them during high-stress seasons or training blocks. The art is to change one major thing at a time so you can feel what's working.

Safety is a design feature when you treat peptides with respect. Start with a qualified medical professional who understands your history, medications, and goals. Align your plan with labs that set baselines and monitor progress—fasting glucose and insulin if you're chasing fat loss, lipids and inflammatory markers if you're rebuilding stamina, thyroid panels if energy has been stubbornly low, and sex-hormone profiles when libido or recovery is the aim. Be conservative on dose; many peptides have a U-shaped curve where "more" delivers less. Watch how you feel first—sleep depth, energy steadiness, training response, mood, digestion—then let labs confirm in the background.

Now, the question almost nobody explains clearly: research-grade peptides versus pharmaceutical-grade peptides. The terms sound similar; the reality is very different. Pharmaceutical grade means the product is manufactured under current Good Manufacturing Practices (cGMP) with validated processes, lot-to-lot consistency, sterility and endotoxin testing, precise potency, stability data, and a documented chain of custody. You can trace the vial in your hand back through a cleanroom to a batch record and a certificate of analysis (COA) tied to that specific lot. For injectables, sterility and endotoxin limits are non-negotiable, and identity/purity are verified by HPLC or mass spectrometry. In short: what the label says is what's in the vial, at the concentration it claims, free of contamination, with a known shelf life.

Research-grade, by contrast, is a catch-all label. It ranges from excellent labs that follow high standards and provide third-party COAs, all the way down to gray-market operations that cut corners on purity, mislabel concentrations, or ship vials with bioburden. The problem isn't that "research-grade" is automatically bad; the problem is that the label tells you almost nothing about quality. This is why source matters so much. If you choose a research-grade product for a peptide that isn't commercially available as a finished drug, work through a medical professional who sources from reputable manufacturers—ideally facilities operating under cGMP-like standards with lot-specific COAs that include identity, purity, potency, and, for injectables, sterility and endotoxin testing.

There's also a legal and ethical layer. Many peptides are not FDA-approved drugs for broad indications; some have approvals in specific contexts, and others are used off-label or compounded by licensed pharmacies under clinician guidance when permitted. Buying from anonymous websites to "save money" introduces risks that dwarf the price difference: dosing errors from inaccurate concentrations, contaminants that inflame tissue or the immune system, and the worst case—something in the vial that isn't what the label says. When your plan depends on sterile, accurately dosed products, the cheapest source is often the most expensive mistake. Partner with a qualified clinician and ask for documentation.

If you need to vet a source, here's a practical script. Ask for a lot-specific certificate of analysis that includes identity testing (MS/HPLC), purity percentage, potency assay, sterility and endotoxin results (if injectable), and a manufacturing date with expiration. Ask whether the facility operates under cGMP or equivalent standards and whether stability testing supports the labeled storage and beyond-use date. If the answers are vague or the documents look generic, walk away. Your health is too valuable to be a chemistry experiment.

Peptides integrate best when the rest of your plan speaks the same language. Pair tissue-healing peptides with a rehab program that progresses load in the direction of your goals. Pair mitochondrial peptides with zone-2 cardio and consistent steps outside. Pair growth-hormone secretagogues with an evening routine that actually allows sleep to happen: earlier dinner, magnesium at night, a cool dark room, and screens off. Pair brain stacks with a task system that protects deep work and daylight breaks so you don't burn the candle at both ends. Pair PT-141 with open conversation and relational time—the molecule can open the door, but you still have to walk through it.

If you're reading this wondering, "Am I missing out by not using peptides?"—the honest answer is that you might be, if you've already put the fundamentals in place and still feel like you're leaving results on the table. For many, peptides are the difference between a program that works on paper and a life that works in practice. The runner whose knees kept her off hills returns to her favorite loop. The founder who woke at 2:30 a.m. thinking about payroll sleeps through and shows up grounded. The new mom finally rebuilds the connective tissue strength pregnancy borrowed from, instead of accepting pain as her new normal. This isn't hype; it's what happens when you amplify the signals your body already recognizes.

Because this field evolves quickly, keep your expectations both high and humble. High, because when you hit the right target, progress feels exponential. Humble, because biology has a pace, and your job is to keep conditions favorable: eat like someone rebuilding tissue, lift like someone who wants to keep doing the activities they love, sleep like it matters, step outside to remind your clock what time it is, and take the supplements that turn enzymes on. When those are in place, peptides do what they're designed to do—create momentum you can feel.

There's a reason more clinicians are adding peptides to the standard BHRT + nutrition + training toolkit: they close the gap between "better" and "this is my life again." If your aim is to walk into your later decades with a body you trust and a mind that's fun to live in, a few well-chosen peptide cycles can be the difference between good and extraordinary. You are not outsourcing your health to a molecule; you are partnering with signals your body already understands to get back what time and stress tried to take.

The future of regenerative medicine isn't one big breakthrough; it's dozens of small, specific instructions delivered at the right time to the right tissue—layered on a foundation of hormones in balance, muscles that do work, food that lowers inflammation, and a nervous system that knows when to be on and when to be off. Peptides are how you speak that language fluently. Used thoughtfully, from reputable sources, inside a plan you can live with, they don't just add years to your life—they add life to your years.

Chapter 9

Gut Health: The Foundation of Wellness

If your body were an orchestra, your gut would be the conductor. Every section—hormones, immunity, brain function, metabolism, mood—takes its timing cues from what happens inside your digestive tract. When that conductor is clear, calm, and coordinated, the music of your health feels effortless. When the gut is inflamed or imbalanced, the entire symphony slips off-beat: energy fades, cravings intensify, sleep frays, hormones misfire, and even your outlook dulls. The good news is that the gut is also one of the fastest systems to heal when given the right inputs. This chapter shows you exactly how to do that, and why gut repair is the leverage point that multiplies the gains you'll see from hormone optimization and peptide therapy.

Think of your gut as both a processing plant and a border—one that has to extract nutrients with incredible precision while blocking unwanted substances. The inside of your small intestine is lined with fingerlike villi carpeted by microscopic microvilli, increasing surface area for absorption. These absorptive cells are joined by "tight junctions," protein gates that should open just enough to pass amino acids, minerals, vitamins, and phytonutrients into circulation—while keeping bacterial fragments, food antigens, and toxins safely inside the tube to be eliminated. When diet, stress, medication exposure, infections, or alcohol loosen these gates, particles slip into the bloodstream and the immune system responds with low-grade, persistent inflammation. The result is the familiar, frustrating set of symptoms many people chalk up to "getting older": bloat, fatigue, brain fog, joint aches, skin flares, and hormone chaos.

Your gut is home to an ecosystem as dense as a rainforest—the microbiome. Trillions of bacteria, viruses, fungi, and archaea live there, training your immune system, fermenting fiber into short-chain fatty acids (SCFAs) like butyrate, and manufacturing vitamins. SCFAs feed your colon cells, help seal the gut barrier, lower inflammation, and even influence gene expression involved in fat burning and insulin sensitivity. When helpful species are crowded out—by ultra-processed foods, chronic stress, alcohol, antibiotics, or low-fiber diets—SCFA production drops, the barrier weakens, and inflammation rises. Restoring diversity through diet, targeted probiotics, and prebiotic fibers is a cornerstone of reclaiming hormonal balance and metabolic flexibility.

The gut and hormones talk constantly. Estrogen metabolism depends on the "estrobolome," a collection of gut microbes that produce enzymes influencing whether estrogen is activated, deactivated, or recirculated. When the estrobolome is out of balance, estrogen can accumulate in forms that worsen PMS, perimenopausal swings, breast tenderness, fibroids, and stubborn midsection weight. Testosterone is also affected by gut inflammation; an inflamed gut increases aromatase activity, pushing testosterone toward excess estrogen in both sexes. Thyroid conversion from T4 to the active T3 occurs substantially in the liver and gut; dysbiosis and a leaky barrier can blunt that conversion, resulting in fatigue, cold intolerance, and slowed metabolism even when a thyroid panel looks "normal." Cortisol, your primary stress hormone, loosens tight junctions and suppresses secretory IgA—the gut's first-line immune coating—making the barrier more permeable and reactive. Heal the gut, and hormone signals get clearer; optimize hormones, and gut lining and motility often improve. This is the virtuous cycle we want to create.

The gut also dictates how your brain feels. Roughly 70% of your immune system surrounds the intestines, and immune messengers from the gut can cross-talk with the brain via the vagus nerve and the bloodstream. Most of your body's serotonin is produced in the gut, and gut bacteria influence the synthesis of GABA and dopamine precursors. When the gut is inflamed, microglia—the brain's immune cells—are more likely to switch into a defensive mode that manifests as brain fog, low motivation, irritability, or anxiety. This is why people often notice that once their gut calms, their thoughts feel brighter and steadier, sleep consolidates, and cravings subside. You're not imagining it—gut-first is brain-first.

How do we restore this system? We use a simple framework: Remove, Replace, Reinoculate, Repair, and Rebalance. First, remove irritants: refined sugar, alcohol for a season, gluten and most grains if you're reactive, industrial seed oils, and ultra-processed foods. Many people run a 21–30-day elimination that also sets aside common triggers like conventional dairy and soy, then reintroduces them one at a time to check tolerance. Second, replace what's missing—stomach acid and digestive enzymes often decline with age and stress, so temporary enzyme support at meals can reduce bloat and improve nutrient extraction. Third, reinoculate with probiotics and prebiotic fibers to restore diversity. Fourth, repair the gut lining with targeted nutrients that feed enterocytes, tighten junctions, and soothe the mucosa. Finally, rebalance stress, sleep, and movement so the improvements stick.

Let's talk about the repair phase because it amplifies every other wellness lever you pull. A comprehensive GI powder can combine the ingredients your lining craves: L-glutamine to fuel intestinal cells; arabinogalactans to support immune balance and beneficial microbe growth; deglycyrrhizinated licorice, slippery elm, and marshmallow to coat and soothe the mucosa; aloe vera to calm inflammation; and zinc-L-carnosine to stabilize the small-bowel lining and stimulate repair. Formulas with this profile are designed to promote regularity, microbial balance, and proper immune function while being gentle enough for daily use in a reset plan.

Immunoglobulin support is another powerful tool when the gut-immune interface is overfiring. Serum-derived immunoglobulins (including IgG) can bind unwanted microbial fragments and dietary antigens in the lumen, preventing their passage across the epithelium and reducing the inflammatory cytokine cascade. This approach helps maintain barrier function without suppressing helpful flora, and may even support athletic recovery by lowering gut-driven immune stress. These powders are typically mixed in water or smoothies and used once or twice daily during a reset.

Probiotics help repopulate and diversify the microbiome—especially when formulas deliver multiple strains with complementary actions and adequate potency. Multi-strain blends around 50 billion CFU commonly include Lactobacillus and Bifidobacterium species that support regularity, urogenital and vaginal health, lactase enzyme production, and gut-lining integrity; some strains like L. salivarius can modulate immune cytokines and adhere well to human epithelial cells. When combined with Streptococcus thermophilus and other partners, these blends cover both small and large intestine niches and help make the gut inhospitable to unwanted organisms. Refrigeration after opening is often recommended for freshness.

Digestive enzymes can be a short-term "training-wheels" solution while the gut heals. Comprehensive blends typically include amylase, lipase, proteases (bromelain, pepsin, trypsin, papain), cellulase, lactase, and sometimes DPP-IV activity to help with gluten fragments. These formulas aim to decrease post-meal fullness, gas, and reflux while improving nutrient absorption. Some combine enzymes with a small probiotic dose and algae-based micronutrients to further support digestion and recovery. Used with meals for 4–12 weeks, they often make a dramatic difference in day-to-day comfort.

From there, we support the microbiome's daily diet. Fiber is not one thing; it's thousands of plant-derived compounds. Non-starchy vegetables, leafy greens, crucifers, herbs, and low-sugar fruits feed beneficial microbes without spiking insulin. Polyphenols in berries, olives, extra virgin olive oil, cacao, green tea, and colorful spices act as prebiotics and antioxidant signals. Clean proteins—from eggs, fish, and ruminants raised on their native diets—provide amino acids for repair. Traditional foods like bone broth offer collagen peptides and minerals that soothe and build the gut lining. The less you rely on ultra-processed foods and seed oils, the faster inflammation calms and the more responsive your hormone receptors become. Many readers notice their BHRT dose works "better" once the gut quiets down; that's receptor sensitivity in action.

The gut reset works even faster when you pair nutrition and nutraceuticals with peptides that directly calm and repair the mucosa. BPC-157—originally isolated from gastric juice—has been widely explored in preclinical and translational settings for its ability to support angiogenesis and tissue healing in the GI tract, tendons, and ligaments. KPV (the C-terminal tripeptide of alpha-MSH) is a potent anti-inflammatory that down-modulates NF-κB signaling and can be used in oral or topical forms to soothe gut and skin flares. Many clinics also use blends that combine BPC-157 with TB4-derived fragments or with KPV in staged protocols during a 6–12 week reset. While peptides are not substitutes for food and lifestyle, they act like an accelerator pedal for repair when used thoughtfully and sourced responsibly through a medical professional.

Because "leaky gut" and dysbiosis can look different from person to person, it's smart to match support to your current state. If you have frequent bloating, alternating constipation and diarrhea, foul gas, and sugar cravings, a practitioner may suspect small intestinal bacterial overgrowth (SIBO) or fungal overgrowth. This is where a time-limited protocol—elimination diet, a temporarily lower-fermentable carbohydrate approach, enzymatic support, targeted probiotics, and, when appropriate, antimicrobial botanicals prescribed by a professional—can reset the terrain. If you're constipated, think motility plus minerals and hydration; if you're loose, think binding, soothing, and calming with GI powders and immunoglobulins. If reflux dominates, look at meal timing, chewing, and enzyme/acid support before assuming you need long-term acid suppression. If your skin is flaring, double down on barrier support and omega-3s while you identify food triggers. Symptom-guided personalization is how you get durable results.

A 28-Day Gut Reset is a practical way to start. In Weeks 1–2, remove common irritants and lower fermentable load if you're very bloated. Begin a comprehensive GI powder daily, add immunoglobulin support once or twice a day, use enzymes with meals, and take a multi-strain probiotic. In Weeks 3–4, continue the core supports, broaden your vegetables and fermented foods as tolerated, and reintroduce one potential trigger every three to four days while tracking mood, sleep, skin, digestion, and energy. Layer in peptides (BPC-157 and/or KPV) for six to eight weeks if your symptoms are moderate to severe or you've had longstanding issues. Keep alcohol minimal during the reset. Walk after meals, sleep seven to nine hours, and practice one simple stress-down ritual daily (nasal breathing, light mobility, or a short nature walk).

As your gut heals, hormone optimization typically becomes smoother. Estrogen detoxification improves, which many women notice as steadier cycles or fewer perimenopausal swings. Thyroid conversion efficiencies rise, so cold hands, low morning energy, and hair shedding can ease. Cortisol swings settle as the body perceives less internal threat, and insulin sensitivity improves along with GLP-1 signaling from a healthier intestinal lining. For men and women, a calmer gut also means less overproduction of aromatase, making it easier to maintain favorable testosterone-to-estrogen balance with therapeutic support. If you've ever felt like your dose of BHRT "suddenly worked," look to the gut—you likely changed something your microbiome loved.

Let's make the protocol tangible. A sample morning might start with water and minerals, a protein-rich breakfast, and your probiotic. If you're using an immunoglobulin powder, mix it in a few ounces of water mid-morning. Take enzymes with lunch and dinner for the first month. Stir your GI repair powder into water in the afternoon when cravings typically strike; the soothing herbs and glutamine often help. If you're on BPC-157 or KPV, take them on a schedule recommended by your practitioner. In the evening, shift to a lower-light environment, eat two to three hours before bed, and prioritize sleep—because the gut lining renews fastest overnight.

Which product categories should you consider in a gut reset? Look for a comprehensive GI repair powder with L-glutamine, arabinogalactans, DGL licorice, aloe 200:1, slippery elm, marshmallow, and zinc-L-carnosine—these ingredients are specifically included to fuel enterocytes, support beneficial bacteria, modulate immune tone, and stabilize mucosal integrity. Add a serum-derived immunoglobulin powder with a standardized content of IgG (often alongside IgA/IgM and transferrin) if your symptoms suggest barrier breakdown or food reactivity. Choose a multi-strain probiotic in the 15–50 billion CFU range with both Lactobacillus and Bifidobacterium species; consider shelf-stable strains if refrigeration is a barrier. Keep a comprehensive digestive enzyme on hand for larger or richer meals. These categories are all represented in professional tech sheets and can be discussed with your clinician to match your situation.

For readers who like to understand the "why" at the ingredient level: L-glutamine is the preferred fuel of intestinal cells and supports villus height. Arabinogalactans (from larch) act as prebiotic fibers and immune modulators, nudging a healthier microbial balance. DGL licorice, slippery elm, and marshmallow lay a protective film over irritated mucosa and have traditional use for reducing bowel transit time and absorbing toxins in the lumen. Aloe 200:1 concentrates the soothing polysaccharides that calm inflammatory signaling. Zinc-L-carnosine complexes zinc with the dipeptide carnosine to target the small bowel lining, stabilizing membrane integrity and stimulating repair. These are the same levers your body pulls on its own—amino acids, minerals, and mucilaginous plant compounds—simply concentrated and combined for therapeutic effect.

What about live microbes? Lactobacillus species help acidify the small intestine and inhibit opportunists; Bifidobacteria favor the colon and produce lactic and acetic acids to crowd out problematic organisms; Streptococcus thermophilus can line the gut wall and, in animal models, reduce airway inflammation after antibiotic exposure. Multi-strain blends work because different strains prefer different neighborhoods in the GI tract and bring distinct benefits—motility support, SCFA production, mucosal adhesion, or immune modulation. This is why many clinicians prefer mixed formulas over single-strain products unless a specific strain is being targeted for a defined purpose.

And enzymes? Aging, stress, and antacid overuse can all reduce digestive secretions. Broad-spectrum enzyme formulas that include amylase, lipase, proteases, lactase, and cellulase—sometimes plus DPP-IV—can help break food down fully so it's less likely to ferment, reflux, or trigger immune reactions. Some blends also include trace minerals and microalgae (spirulina/chlorella) to supply co-factors and gentle antioxidant support. Use them with meals for a season, then taper as your own digestion improves.

Safety matters. Choose professional-grade products, especially for immunoglobulins and probiotics where potency and purity are crucial. For peptides, source under medical supervision. If you're pregnant, nursing, on immunosuppressants, or have significant GI disease (IBD, celiac disease, active ulcers), work with a knowledgeable clinician to personalize your protocol. Remember that "more" is not always "better"; the goal is to restore balance, not overwhelm your system with a dozen new inputs overnight.

Two brief snapshots from practice show what's possible. A 45-year-old woman with perimenopausal swings, cystic acne, and bloating began an elimination plan plus GI repair powder, immunoglobulins twice daily, a multi-strain probiotic, and enzymes with meals. Within six weeks her skin calmed, sleep consolidated, and her cycle symptoms stabilized; later, when she added hormone optimization, a modest dose went further than expected. A 58-year-old man with reflux and joint aches reduced alcohol, removed gluten, used enzymes and a GI powder, took probiotics and omega-3s, and added BPC-157 for eight weeks. His reflux eased enough to taper off acid-suppressing medication (with his physician's guidance), joint stiffness improved, and he resumed strength training without setbacks. Different stories, same pattern: fix the gut, and everything else gets easier.

Finally, keep what you gain. Eat mostly real, unprocessed food rich in fiber and polyphenols. Hydrate. Walk after meals. Strength train a couple of days a week, breathe through your nose during easy cardio, and go to bed on a schedule. Manage stress so cortisol doesn't undo your hard work. Revisit probiotics for a month after travel or antibiotics. Keep a GI repair powder and a digestive enzyme on hand for seasons of higher stress or when you know your meals will be heavier. Keep listening to your gut—literally and figuratively. It will tell you what's working.

When your gut and hormones are aligned, you don't just feel "fine"—you feel capable. You make sharper decisions, recover faster, and savor your days more fully. That is the real foundation of longevity: a resilient gut ecology, a sturdy barrier, clear hormone signaling, high mitochondrial output, and a calm, focused mind. Build your reset with food, strategically selected nutraceuticals, and, when appropriate, peptides—and watch how quickly your body remembers what vibrant feels like.

Chapter 10

Cellular Health & Mitochondrial Function

If your cells were cities, mitochondria would be the power plants that keep the lights on, the trains running, and the streets safe. When those power plants hum, you feel it everywhere: steady energy from morning to night, clear thinking, better workouts, deeper sleep, and a mood that doesn't wobble with every stressor. When they sputter, you feel that too: afternoon crashes, brain fog, stubborn weight, creaky joints, slower recovery, and a sense that your "battery" doesn't hold a charge like it used to. Mitochondria aren't a fringe topic for biohackers; they're the foundation of healthy aging. Modern longevity science even lists mitochondrial dysfunction among the central hallmarks of aging—a hub that interacts with inflammation, epigenetic drift, and impaired cellular cleanup. The liberating message of this chapter is simple: you can rebuild mitochondrial capacity at any age, and when you do, every other system—from hormones to metabolism to brain performance—becomes easier to optimize.

To appreciate why mitochondria matter, let's zoom in. Each mitochondrion houses an elegant conveyor belt called the electron transport chain (ETC). Electrons travel down this chain, past a series of protein complexes embedded in the inner mitochondrial membrane, and the cell captures their energy to make adenosine triphosphate (ATP)—the fuel that powers every heartbeat, thought, and muscle contraction. As a byproduct, mitochondria also generate tiny pulses of reactive oxygen species (ROS). In the right dose and rhythm, these ROS act like a training signal, nudging cells to build sturdier membranes and antioxidant defenses, and even to create brand-new mitochondria. In excess, ROS become "noise," damaging proteins and DNA. Mitochondrial health is largely about keeping that signal-to-noise ratio right: enough challenge to adapt, not so much that the system frays.

Your body actively manages mitochondrial quality. It builds new ones (biogenesis), recycles damaged ones (mitophagy), and constantly reshapes them via fission and fusion to meet changing demand. A master coordinator called PGC-1α helps open the blueprints for making more and better mitochondria. With age, chronic stress, poor sleep, and ultraprocessed food, PGC-1α signaling tends to drop, mitochondrial turnover slows, and the power grid of your body becomes brittle. The empowering truth is that you can re-engage this machinery with specific levers: training, sleep, nutrient density, stress control, and—when appropriate—BHRT, peptides, and targeted nutraceuticals that support the electron transport chain and membrane resilience.

Training is the most reliable "language" mitochondria understand. Brief, repeated efforts that raise your heart rate—think 30–60 seconds of fast uphill walking or cycling followed by easy recovery—upregulate PGC-1α and mitochondrial protein content, particularly in older adults who start out more depleted. Steady, conversational-pace movement raises your total mitochondrial "bank" and improves fat-burning efficiency. Resistance training may not always enlarge mitochondria directly, but it increases muscle quality, insulin sensitivity, and the metabolic sink that offloads glucose and fats—indirect wins that protect your power plants. In practice, a blend works best: two short interval sessions, two strength sessions, and easy movement most other days. Scale the effort to your starting point and recovery capacity.

Sleep is where these adaptations "take." At night, mitochondria repair lipid membranes, tidy up damaged components, and restock antioxidant systems. Even partial sleep loss raises oxidative stress and blunts next-day energy. If you're training and eating well but still dragging, audit the basics: a consistent bedtime, a darker/cooler room, and fewer screens late. These aren't just nice habits—they're mitochondrial therapy. As sleep regularizes, energy and mood often lift before your labs even change.

Nutrition is your daily vote for or against mitochondrial resilience. Your power plants love steady access to B vitamins, magnesium, iron, copper, selenium, omega-3 fatty acids, and amino acids. They suffer with spikes—blood sugar surges, alcohol binges, or industrial seed oils that make membranes rigid and prone to oxidative wear. Start simple: anchor meals with high-quality protein, cover your plate with low-glycemic vegetables and herbs rich in polyphenols, use extra virgin olive oil and omega-3-rich fish regularly, and match starch portions to activity. These patterns lower inflammation, stabilize insulin, and sharpen mitochondrial signaling. Over time, they even nudge gene expression toward better fat-burning and antioxidant capacity.

Hormones are the system-level dial that helps mitochondria meet demand. Thyroid hormone (especially T3) directly regulates mitochondrial activity and biogenesis—it literally tells cells to build more "power plants." Testosterone supports muscle protein synthesis and mitochondrial density through mechanical loading, while estrogen improves mitochondrial efficiency, antioxidant defenses, and cerebral blood flow. When these hormones slide below optimal, trying to upgrade your cellular grid can feel like renovating a building while the power keeps brown-out levels. This is why properly tailored Bioidentical Hormone Replacement Therapy (BHRT) can be a force multiplier for energy. Correcting thyroid under-conversion, restoring estrogen and progesterone balance in women, and re-establishing physiologic testosterone in both sexes creates a cellular environment that finally responds to smart training and nutrition.

Peptides give you a precision toolkit. MOTS-C—a mitochondrial-derived peptide—helps cells handle metabolic stress by engaging the folate–AICAR–AMPK pathway. In early human and translational research, MOTS-C has been associated with better glucose handling, improved stamina under stress, and signals tied to healthy aging. Some programs pair MOTS-C with AICAR (an AMPK activator used in research settings) to raise "cellular idle," making it easier to move more and burn cleaner, especially when layered onto protein-forward, low-inflammatory eating. These tools should be sourced through reputable medical channels for quality, identity, and dosing assurance—and they work best as accelerators alongside sleep, movement, and nutrition, not as substitutes.

Now let's zoom into two powerhouse nutraceuticals that directly support mitochondrial output—and that pair beautifully with the lifestyle, BHRT, and peptide levers above.

EnerCoQ10 is centered on coenzyme Q10 (CoQ10), the shuttle molecule that ferries electrons inside the ETC and helps stabilize mitochondrial membranes. Because high-energy tissues like heart, brain, and muscle are packed with mitochondria, they are especially sensitive to CoQ10 sufficiency. The EnerCoQ10 professional sheet highlights CoQ10's role in ATP formation and antioxidant defense, and notes that certain medications—especially cholesterol-lowering drugs—may reduce CoQ10 status or increase need, contributing to fatigue or muscle discomfort in some individuals. Their suggested intake range for adults commonly runs 100–300 mg per day under practitioner guidance, with a chewable wafer providing 300 mg CoQ10 per serving. Here's what makes this formula distinctive for mitochondrial care: alongside CoQ10, each chewable includes vitamin E (a membrane-protective antioxidant) and 300 mg of DMG (more on DMG in a moment), creating a stack that supports electron flow, protects lipid membranes, and may improve oxygen handling and circulation—all practical wins for people rebuilding their energy system.*

EnerDMG focuses on N,N-dimethylglycine (DMG), an adaptogenic nutrient with a surprisingly wide reach. As an indirect methyl donor, DMG contributes "one-carbon" units to reactions involved in synthesizing neurotransmitters, antibodies, nucleic acids, and hormones—many of the parts your cells need to build and repair. The EnerDMG sheet summarizes research and clinician experience suggesting DMG may support physical and mental performance, oxygen utilization, immune balance (including antibody and cytokine production), vascular health, and healthy glucose and fat metabolism. Mechanistically, DMG appears to help cells use oxygen more efficiently during stress and exercise, reducing lactic acid buildup and perceived fatigue. In practice, this can translate to steadier energy, better endurance at a given workload, and clearer focus when demands stack up. Because mitochondrial function is tightly coupled to oxygen management and redox balance, DMG becomes a logical ally in any energy-restoration program.*

A smart way to combine these is to use EnerCoQ10 as a daily ETC "wiring and antioxidant" support and layer EnerDMG for periods of higher cognitive or physical demand, or during structured training blocks. Some practitioners prefer daily DMG use in individuals with high workload and immune stress, while others cycle it around peak demands. Either way, the pair addresses both the hardware (ETC electron transport and membrane stability) and the software (methylation-dependent synthesis and oxygen handling) of mitochondrial output.

Did you know? Many human cells contain **hundreds** of mitochondria, and the highest-energy organs—brain, heart, skeletal muscle—are absolutely packed with them. That's one reason changes in mitochondrial fitness are felt first as shifts in mental clarity, exercise capacity, and day-long stamina. *

So how do you build a mitochondria-first day that integrates these tools without becoming a second job? Start with a morning routine that exposes you to natural light and some gentle movement, then eat a protein-anchored breakfast within the first couple of hours of waking. On two non-consecutive days each week, do 10–20 minutes of intervals: a warm-up, 6–8 rounds of 30–60 seconds hard / equal easy, and a cool-down. Add two short full-body strength sessions built around pushes, pulls, hinges, and squats. Walk on most of the in-between days. Aim for 7–9 hours of relatively consistent sleep in a dark, cool room. Eat mostly unprocessed, fiber-rich foods and scale starches to activity. If your symptoms and labs suggest, talk with a qualified provider about BHRT; when hormones are optimized, training and nutrition gains "stick." Consider EnerCoQ10 as a base mitochondrial support and EnerDMG to enhance oxygen use and stress resilience, especially on interval or long workdays. If your clinician includes peptides, a MOTS-C protocol may be layered in cycles to reinforce AMPK-driven adaptations.

Safety and sourcing matter. Work with a clinician for hormone and peptide protocols, especially if you have medical conditions or take prescriptions. Obtain peptides through reputable medical channels that verify identity and purity. Choose professional-grade nutraceuticals with third-party testing. Remember that no supplement replaces the fundamentals—they multiply them. The heavy lifters for mitochondria will always be sleep, movement, nutrient-dense food, and (when indicated) restoration of hormone signaling—while targeted products like EnerCoQ10, EnerDMG, magnesium, omega-3s, and a methylated B complex close critical gaps so your cellular power plants can actually keep up with demand.*

Two brief snapshots show what this looks like in real life. A 62-year-old woman with "I do everything right" fatigue, evening brain fog, and poor workout recovery discovered borderline low thyroid function and menopausal estrogen decline. After optimizing hormones and building a training rhythm of two interval and two strength sessions per week, she added a daily CoQ10-based mitochondrial stack and cycled DMG around work sprints. Within four weeks, she noticed fewer crashes; by eight weeks, deeper sleep and consistent training logs; by six months, a measurable uptick in VO_2-related metrics and a revitalized steady energy she hadn't felt in years. A 55-year-old man with abdominal weight, afternoon slumps, and "wired-tired" nights started with a gut reset to reduce inflammation, then introduced a mitochondria-focused plan: time-consistent sleep, protein-forward eating, EnerCoQ10 daily, EnerDMG on training days, and a supervised MOTS-C cycle. As his non-exercise movement rose and evening meals moved earlier, his waist dropped, insulin resistance markers improved, and he described his days as "quietly energized" rather than up-and-down. Different stories, same pattern: restore the grid and everything else runs better.

A practical weekly blueprint helps these choices become automatic. Monday: intervals + EnerDMG in the late morning, EnerCoQ10 with breakfast. Tuesday: easy walk and mobility. Wednesday: strength (45 minutes, full-body) + consistent protein and colorful plants. Thursday: intervals again, early dinner, lights down. Friday: strength + longer evening walk. Saturday: leisure movement—hike, bike, play—with family or friends. Sunday: reset—prep a few protein and veggie staples, set bed/wake times, review labs or training notes every 4–8 weeks to adjust. If work or travel spikes, keep the "non-negotiables": sleep window, protein at breakfast, and your mitochondria stack. Consistency beats intensity.

Finally, align expectations with biology. Mitochondria respond fast to good inputs—some adaptations begin within days—but durable change is measured in weeks and months as your cells build new hardware. You don't have to be perfect; you have to be consistent. Each night of good sleep, each protein-anchored meal, each bout of smart training, each decision to step outside, is a vote for more capacity. Layer BHRT thoughtfully when indicated, use peptides and nutraceuticals to accelerate repair and close gaps, and keep tailoring the plan to your season of life. This is how you build a body that feels younger than your birthdate suggests—not with shortcuts, but by restoring the cellular machinery that powers everything you care to do.

*Professional sheets for EnerCoQ10 and EnerDMG describe these roles in accessible language and provide suggested serving information for practitioner-guided use. Always consult your healthcare provider for personalized advice.

Chapter 11

Exercise & Strength Training for Longevity

Muscle is the quiet hero of healthy aging, the load-bearing wall in the house of your body that most people don't notice until it starts to thin. You feel its presence in a thousand ordinary ways—when you rise from the floor without planning a strategy, when you hoist a carry-on into the overhead bin without holding your breath, when a missed night of sleep doesn't derail the whole week because your system has reserves. You also feel its absence—stairs that ask too many questions, jars that require negotiation, afternoons that slide into fog. Strength training changes that trajectory. Not because you're chasing a look, but because every repetition is a message to your physiology: build, repair, get ready for more life.

If you strip away the noise of fitness trends, the principle is simple: your body adapts to what you ask of it. Ask little, and it obliges by becoming economical and conservative. Ask for strength and power, and it reorganizes to deliver—adding contractile tissue, thickening tendons, making bones more resilient, upgrading the mitochondria that turn food and oxygen into energy. Those upgrades reach far beyond the mirror. Blood sugar steadies because muscle is the largest sink for glucose in the body. Sleep deepens because training helps align your circadian rhythm and increases the "pressure" for restorative rest. Mood stabilizes because muscles release anti-inflammatory signals (myokines) that talk directly to your brain. Even confidence improves, not as an abstract idea but as the physical recognition that your body says yes when life asks for effort.

There's a profound partnership between hormones and training. When sex hormones live in functional ranges, the same workout produces more muscle and less soreness. When thyroid conversion is healthy, the work you put in feels proportional to the results you get back. When cortisol rises in the morning and falls at night instead of flattening all day, motivation shows up when you need it and recovery shows up when you deserve it. Optimized hormones don't replace training; they let your training "stick." And the relationship runs both directions. Strength work improves insulin sensitivity, which makes sex-hormone signaling cleaner. Better sleep after a training day improves thyroid conversion. Calmer baseline inflammation makes receptors listen more closely to the signals you're restoring. This is why a sane movement plan is a pillar of longevity rather than an optional hobby.

Most people don't need a complicated program or endless hours in a gym. They need enough signal to force adaptation and enough recovery to let it happen. Two or three focused strength sessions in a week, paired with frequent easy movement on the other days, is a minimum that matters. Choose big human patterns your body already understands—squatting and standing, hinging at the hips, pushing and pulling, lunging and carrying. Use tools that fit your world: dumbbells in the guest room, kettlebells in the garage, a cable machine at the community center, bodyweight and a park bench on a good day outside. What matters is progression. If last month's weight feels exactly the same this month, nothing meaningful is changing. If form degrades just to move the load, you're not progressing; you're performing. Progression lives in the quiet details—one more perfect rep, a few more pounds handled crisply, a steadier tempo through the lowering phase, a shorter rest interval while technique stays sharp.

You don't have to memorize rep charts to train intelligently. Think in broad zones. Heavier, lower-rep work teaches your nervous system to recruit fibers and tells bone to stay dense. Moderate rep ranges with controlled tempos are where a lot of muscle is built and metabolic health improves. Higher-rep, slow-lowering sets are friendly to tendons and teach joints to tolerate load through full range. Sprinkle in brief, well-rested bursts of speed—a few medicine-ball throws, some crisp kettlebell swings after coaching, short hill strides on a walk—to remind your fast-twitch fibers they still exist. Rotate those emphases across the month. Your tissues don't need the same lesson every session, and your brain appreciates novelty with purpose.

Cardiovascular health thrives on two simple ingredients: lots of easy movement and a small amount of hard movement. The easy piece is a pace where you can breathe through your nose and talk in short sentences—brisk walks, gentle cycling, relaxed laps in a pool. Do that most days, even if it's spread in ten-minute slices around your schedule. The hard piece is short for you, not for an athlete on television—fifteen to thirty seconds of effort that feels fast at your current fitness, followed by equal easy time to recover, repeated a handful of times after a warm-up and before a cool-down. One short session like that each week keeps capacity you will be grateful to have when real life asks you to move quickly. Overdo the hard stuff and you strangle recovery; underdo it and you lose the ability to respond when it matters. The middle—endlessly "kinda hard"—is where many people spin their wheels and wonder why they're tired without getting fitter.

Mobility doesn't require an hour of elaborate routines. It benefits from restoring the motions you're about to use. Before lower-body work, spend a couple minutes coaxing ankles forward toward a wall, prying the hips gently through rotation, waking up hamstrings with controlled slides. Before upper-body work, open the mid-back with easy book-openers, set your shoulder blades with band pull-aparts and hanging shrugs, rehearse external rotation so pressing and pulling feel centered. Afterward, walk slowly and breathe through your nose with a longer exhale than inhale for a few minutes. That tells your nervous system it's safe to leave "go mode" and invest in recovery. Tendons respond beautifully to slow loading; if your elbows, Achilles, or patellar tendon grumble, include sets where you lower the weight for a deliberate count and pause without bouncing before you rise. Do that a couple times a week for several weeks, and those tissues often become quieter travel companions.

Recovery is where the magic lands. Training is the signal. Food, sleep, and targeted support are the construction crew. Aim for protein at each meal—not as punishment, but as the raw material for everything you're trying to build. A helpful target for active adults reclaiming strength is roughly 1.6 to 2.0 grams of protein per kilogram of body weight per day, spread across meals your schedule will actually allow. Fill the rest of the plate with colorful plants, herbs, and low-glycemic starches sized to your activity. Those polyphenols and fibers calm inflammatory noise and feed a gut that absorbs what you eat. Keep alcohol modest, especially late. Nothing wrecks sleep architecture and next-day power like a couple of innocent drinks at the wrong time. Treat bedtime like an appointment with tomorrow's clarity—dim lights, cool room, familiar wind-down, devices asleep before you are.

When foundations are in motion, targeted nutraceuticals can remove bottlenecks. An evidence-informed omega-3 supports joints and blood vessels that you're asking to work. A methylated B complex can smooth energy output on higher-demand weeks. Balanced vitamins A, D3, and K2 help bones and vasculature use minerals wisely and keep hormone receptors listening. Magnesium is a quiet hero for muscle relaxation and deeper sleep, especially in well-absorbed forms taken in the evening. Comprehensive mineral blends with zinc and selenium support repair enzymes and hormone signaling. If training makes sluggish thyroid conversion obvious—cold hands, flat energy despite effort—a comprehensive thyroid support that includes nutrients like selenium and iron sufficiency, with iodine when appropriate, helps the signal reach your cells. These aren't replacements for food or sleep; they're levers that make adaptation easier.

Peptides are not shortcuts; they are specific nudges to systems you're actively engaging. If long-standing connective tissue complaints have been the reason you avoid training, a tissue-healing signal like BPC-157 can support tendon and ligament remodeling while also helping the gut absorb the nutrition your plan depends on. If you're rebuilding sleep depth as you reintroduce strength work, a short, clinician-guided course of growth-hormone secretagogues such as CJC-1295 with Ipamorelin can deepen slow-wave sleep and shorten the distance between lights-out and real rest—improving next-day recovery more than any gadget. If aerobic capacity is your weak link, mitochondrial-focused nudges like MOTS-C, sometimes cycled with other AMPK-engaging tools under professional supervision, can help cells handle metabolic stress so sessions feel "doable" sooner. In select, supervised cases where muscle protein synthesis is especially stubborn, targeted IGF-1 protocols are layered alongside appropriate protein and mechanical tension. These tools are always adjuncts; they multiply the returns on smart training, honest nutrition, and protected sleep. Quality and sourcing matter—work with a qualified clinician and insist on identity and purity assurance.

One of the most empowering realities about training is that it's adaptable to every season of life and every hormonal chapter. Perimenopause and menopause don't sideline you; they change your playbook. You may need longer warm-ups, slightly fewer weekly sets, and a higher protein target to get the same response you saw in your thirties. Sleep becomes your amplifier—protect it and everything improves. If hot flashes or night wakings are chewing through recovery, that's a signal to stabilize hormones, calm the nervous system, and then let training cash those checks. Andropause brings its own pattern; the plan is similar: keep intensity, manage volume, protect sleep, and expose your muscles to regular, meaningful load. When sex hormones and thyroid are tuned, you'll notice the difference quickly: the same session produces more progress and less soreness. When they aren't, training exposes gaps—persistent fatigue, inexplicable plateaus, soreness out of proportion to the work. Use that feedback to adjust the bigger plan with your provider.

It's helpful to track metrics that predict independence rather than obsess over the scale. Notice how your grip strength changes as you lift consistently; it's a surprisingly strong predictor of resilience. Time how fast you can sit down in a chair and stand up five times without using your hands; that simple test reflects leg strength, balance, and coordination you use daily. Pay attention to how far you can carry two moderate objects in one minute without setting them down; life is full of carries. Practice single-leg balance while you brush your teeth and watch it improve across weeks; that skill is an anti-fall vaccine. And measure your walking pace on a loop you enjoy; the ease of your "easy pace" is one of the quietest signs you're getting younger from the inside out.

You might be wondering how to begin if it's been years. Start smaller than your ambition. Two thirty-minute full-body sessions per week are enough to change your life if you keep showing up. Pick five movements you can perform well: sit-to-stands from a box, a hip hinge with a light weight held close, an incline push-up against a counter, a supported row with a band or dumbbell, and a walk with something in your hands that asks your grip to participate. Do two sets of eight to twelve crisp reps, leave a couple of reps in the tank, and add a tiny bit next week. Walk ten minutes after dinner. After four weeks, add a third set to the first two movements. After eight, add a few playful throws with a light medicine ball, or hike a hill you've been avoiding. Momentum is the point; heroics are optional.

If you already walk but never lift, keep your walks and add two strength sessions. Goblet squats, Romanian deadlifts, one-arm rows, overhead presses that don't pinch, and suitcase carries are a complete education. Start in the middle rep ranges, feel the muscles you're training instead of just finishing the numbers, and add something—one rep, a little weight, a calmer tempo—each week. Replace one steady walk with a short "spark" session: six brief hill strides with easy returns. Your heart and lungs will thank you without asking you to become a runner.

If you lift and feel stuck, you might be recovered enough to train but not recovered enough to adapt. Trim the junk volume that exists only to tire you out. Make your first lift truly heavy for a few clean sets, follow with moderate rep ranges where you feel tension and control, and finish with one higher-rep set that's kind to tendons. Plan a lighter week every fourth week where you do the same moves with 60–

70% of the usual load and walk out feeling better than you walked in. Log your work; progress you can see is easier to believe.

If your joints are skeptical, train around pain, not through it. Swap deep squats for box squats at a comfortable height while you rebuild tolerance. Use trap-bar deadlifts or hip thrusts if your back protests conventional deadlifts. Row more than you press overhead until the shoulders glide again. Strengthen calves and feet; a lot of "knee pain" starts at the ankle. Add slow-lowering calf raises and pay attention to how much easier stairs feel in a month.

Balance and power deserve specific attention because falls aren't random—they're the end of a long, quiet slide in strength, reflexes, and proprioception. Practice getting up and down from the floor in different ways. Include carries in every week: farmer's (both hands), suitcase (one hand), and rack (weights at chest height). Those patterns teach your core to resist unwanted motion while your hips do the work—exactly what life asks of you when you carry groceries, a child, or a suitcase. Add a few crisp throws against a wall or into open space with full rest between efforts. The goal is not fatigue; it's speed of intent.

Rucking is an elegant bridge for people who prefer fresh air to fluorescent lights. Put a modest weight in a backpack—ten to fifteen percent of your body weight is plenty at the start—and walk a familiar loop with good posture. It's strength and cardio in one practice, it asks your grip and core to participate, and it sneaks resilience into your week without requiring a membership. Rowing machines are joint-friendly teachers of rhythm and power if you keep your posture honest. A playground can be a full gym: step-ups on a low bench, push-ups at an incline, rows hanging from a bar, easy hangs to open your shoulders. The best program is the one you will do.

Common fears are worth answering out loud. You won't "get bulky" by accident. That body type lives at the intersection of uncommon genetics, unusual volume, and deliberate intent. What you will get is muscle that makes clothes fit better, backs complain less, and appetites behave. "Bad knees" are often undertrained knees connected to stiff ankles and weak hips. Strength built thoughtfully is one of the kindest things you can do for them. "No time" is real—so is the reality that ten minutes three times a day beats zero. Two sets of squats, two sets of rows, a one-minute carry, and a brisk walk are enough to move the needle. "Too old to start" dissolves in front of the evidence; people well into their eighties add strength and function with progressive resistance. Start smaller, progress slower, celebrate the wins.

It helps to imagine a few real lives. A creative director in her mid-forties arrived wired-tired from years of late nights and urgent deliverables. She began with two thirty-minute sessions each week: goblet squats, hip hinges with a kettlebell, incline push-ups, one-arm rows, loaded carries. She walked after dinner and protected sleep like a deadline. Four weeks later, her resting heart rate dropped and her three-o'clock fog loosened. By eight weeks, she added a short hill-stride session and noticed her mood didn't fray by late afternoon. Twelve weeks in, her carry distance doubled, her calendar felt less predatory, and the mirror changed as a side effect rather than the goal. A contractor nearing sixty assumed lifting would aggravate his back and elbows. Instead, he learned to hinge, brace, and pull with his lats. Trap-bar deadlifts replaced awkward bending at work, slow eccentrics quieted his elbow, and two days a week of thoughtful strength made his job feel less like attrition. After twelve weeks, he slept without hot spots, carried more comfortably on site, and saw labs that moved in the right direction. A retired teacher in her early sixties feared falling more than anything. Her plan emphasized balance and power she hadn't asked for in years: sit-to-stands, step-downs, medicine-ball chest passes, suitcase carries, daily walking. With hormones stabilized earlier and sleep now a priority, training paid immediate dividends. Three months later she could get off the floor without planning. Six months later she booked a hiking trip she'd talked herself out of for years.

Training integrates with everything else you've learned in this book. When hormones are tuned, lean mass returns more quickly and recovery feels satisfying instead of punitive. When the gut is healthier, you actually absorb the protein and minerals your muscles crave. When sleep is honest, strength shows up on schedule. If your plan includes targeted nutraceuticals, choose them with intention—omega-3s to soften inflammatory edges, ADK-style support to shepherd minerals into bone, magnesium to deepen rest, a methylated B complex to support energy in high-demand seasons, comprehensive minerals to keep cramps at bay, thyroid cofactors when signs point to sluggish conversion. If peptide support is on the table with your clinician, use it strategically—around the start of a new program, a return from injury, or a planned push—not as a permanent crutch. The story is always the same: training supplies the signal, your internal environment determines how loudly your body hears it.

Did you know? Skeletal muscle is the largest glucose sink in your body. The more of it you keep and the more of it you use, the easier it is to maintain steady energy, tame cravings, and age with a metabolism that cooperates.

A dozen weeks is enough to notice meaningful change. The first month is about grooves and positions—learning how a squat feels in your hips and ankles, how a hinge feels in your hamstrings and glutes, how a row feels in your back rather than your neck. The second month adds progression and a small touch of speed—weights that inch up, reps that accrue, a medicine-ball throw that feels surprisingly fun. The third month introduces heavier sets for your first lift and moderate, controlled work for the rest, with a lighter deload week at the end so your body cashes the checks you've been writing. Across those weeks, your "easy pace" gets easier, your sleep acquires weight, and the way you inhabit your day changes first before any number does.

If there's a mindset that makes this all stick, it's to love what the training gives you more than the training itself. Love the feeling of carrying all the groceries in one trip, of getting up from the floor without thinking, of hiking a hill without bargaining, of feeling your brain operate at full brightness at three in the afternoon. Log your sessions so progress has a place to live. Be politely stubborn about sleep.

Eat like someone rebuilding tissue. Let strength be the vote you cast against frailty every week you're alive.

Decline is not a straight line etched into your birth certificate; it's a slope influenced by choices that add up. Strength training is one of the most reliable levers you can pull to change that slope. When you pair it with an internal environment that listens—hormones in range, inflammation quieted, nutrients available, sleep respected—your body will surprise you with how fast it remembers. Getting older is a given. Getting weaker is a choice. Choose a future where your body keeps saying yes.

Chapter 12

Nutrition for Longevity & Hormonal Health

How Food Signals and Core Nutrients Shape Hormones, Metabolism, and Healthy Aging

Food is more than calories; it is a language your cells understand. Every meal delivers signals that nudge physiology toward repair or wear, clarity or fog, leanness or storage. When those signals are consistent—protein anchored, colorful plants abundant, fats chosen wisely, and meals spaced so digestion can finish—you feel it as steadier energy, deeper sleep, better training response, and a mood that holds its ground. When the signals are chaotic—ultra-processed products, grazing all day, sugar spikes, late-night overeating—your body reads stress and answers with cravings, inflammation, and hormonal static. The solution is not a crash diet; it is a pattern that keeps your biochemistry on your side, and it pairs naturally with BHRT and peptides so all three work in concert.

A practical way to think about nutrition is as the operating system for hormone sensitivity. Protein supplies amino acids for enzymes, neurotransmitters, and the hormones themselves. Healthy fats build cell membranes and the steroid backbone of estrogen, progesterone, testosterone, and cortisol. Low-glycemic carbohydrates from vegetables, legumes, roots, and modest fruit replenish glycogen without shouting at insulin. Micronutrients act like software updates that keep the system responsive. Put those pieces together and the signals from optimized hormones land cleanly, while peptide protocols for repair and mitochondrial efficiency gain traction.

Insulin is the first signal most modern lives need to calm. It is designed to store energy, not to rule metabolism all day. You improve insulin sensitivity with protein-forward meals; plenty of non-starchy vegetables; unrefined fats that slow gastric emptying; and starch portions scaled to activity. A breakfast centered on eggs, fish, meat, Greek-style yogurt, or a clean protein shake—and paired with fiber like chia, flax, or berries—quietly sets up your entire day. From there, think "fiber + color" at every meal: polyphenol-rich plants act as mild hormetic stressors that upregulate antioxidant defenses and improve cellular signaling, including how well your cells "hear" insulin.

Protein deserves its own paragraph. With age we develop anabolic resistance, meaning muscles need a clearer nudge to build. Cross the leucine threshold at each meal—usually 25–45 grams of high-quality protein depending on body size—and distribute intake across the day. Animal proteins (eggs, poultry, ruminant meats, dairy where tolerated, and seafood) and well-constructed plant combinations (legumes plus seeds/grains) provide the essential amino acids your tissues require. Pair protein with resistance training and you restore two of the strongest longevity levers: muscle mass and insulin sensitivity.

Fats are structural allies, not villains. Prioritize extra-virgin olive oil, avocado, nuts, seeds, pasture-raised egg yolks, and coconut for their monounsaturated and saturated profiles that stabilize membranes and support hormone synthesis. Use concentrated omega-3 fatty acids (EPA and DHA) from cold-water fish or a purified marine oil to lower inflammatory signaling and support cardiovascular and brain health. The fats to limit are industrial seed oils common in packaged foods and deep-fryers; their fragile fatty acids and oxidation byproducts can amplify inflammation and disrupt membrane function.

Carbohydrates are tools. Non-starchy plants should carry most of the daily load, with starchy roots, tubers, and properly prepared grains used according to activity levels. Many people do well placing the majority of starch around training or earlier in the day, and avoiding heavy late-night carb loads that fragment sleep. If mid-section fat, cravings, and afternoon slumps are a theme, try a "carb back-control" approach: protein and vegetables dominate breakfast and lunch; a modest starch portion is reserved for dinner on training days.

Micronutrients keep all of this working. Vitamin D acts like a hormone, influencing immunity, insulin sensitivity, bone turnover, and mood; aim to keep blood levels in an optimal range confirmed by labs. Vitamin K2 (especially MK-7) directs calcium toward bone and away from arteries, while vitamin A supports epithelial integrity and healthy receptor function. Together, vitamins A/D3/K2 form a trio that strengthens bones and clarifies hormone signaling. Methylated B vitamins (methylfolate, methylcobalamin, P-5-P) drive methylation reactions crucial for neurotransmitter balance and estrogen detoxification and help keep homocysteine in check. Magnesium—ideally as well-tolerated forms such as glycinate, malate, or threonate—supports hundreds of reactions, improving sleep depth, muscle relaxation, and glucose control. Essential minerals like selenium, zinc, and iodine (when appropriate) support thyroid conversion from T4 to T3; iron sufficiency prevents fatigue and hair loss; copper, manganese, and molybdenum serve antioxidant enzymes and connective tissue.

Your gut decides whether any of this reaches its destination. The intestinal lining is a selectively permeable barrier; the microbiome metabolizes fiber into short-chain fatty acids that cool inflammation, strengthen the barrier, and influence estrogen metabolism through the estrobolome. When the estrobolome is balanced, estrogen metabolites trend toward brain-, bone-, and vessel-friendly forms; when it's disrupted, symptoms escalate. You support this ecosystem with diverse fibers (leafy greens, brassicas, onions, garlic, asparagus, berries), fermented foods as tolerated, mindful chewing, and meal spacing that leaves time for the migrating motor complex to "sweep" the small intestine between meals.

When the gut is reactive—after antibiotics, infections, alcohol, significant stress, or years of ultra-processed food—targeted support accelerates repair. Immunoglobulin G concentrates bind microbial antigens and toxins in the lumen so they can be escorted out of the body. Broad-spectrum botanical protocols (for example, combinations including berberine, oregano extract, allicin, caprylic acid, and pau d'arco) help reduce bacterial and yeast overgrowths documented by history or testing. If parasites are suspected, practitioner-guided botanical formulas can be used short-term. Once the microbial burden is lowered, mucosal-support nutrients—L-glutamine, zinc carnosine, aloe vera, deglycyrrhizinated licorice (DGL), N-acetyl-glucosamine, and slippery elm—help rebuild the barrier so absorption improves and immune noise quiets.

Now link nutrition to hormones you can feel. Stable glucose and insulin make thyroid, estrogen, progesterone, and testosterone signals easier for cells to interpret. Magnesium enhances progesterone's calming nighttime effect. Omega-3 intake reduces inflammatory "static," improving receptor responsiveness. Adequate protein plus strength training naturally boosts satiety hormones and preserves lean mass. A/D/K2 supports bone and vascular health in estrogen- and testosterone-supported bodies. Diindolylmethane (DIM), from cruciferous vegetables or a purified supplement, nudges estrogen toward favorable metabolites. And a calm gut microbiome prevents excessive recirculation of hormonally active compounds.

Time matters. A 10–12-hour eating window most days respects circadian biology, improves glycemic control, and supports sleep. Leave roughly three hours between the last bite and bedtime. If you train early, include protein within an hour of finishing; if training is late afternoon, make dinner protein-forward and keep starch purposeful, not automatic.

Hydration quietly sets the stage for focus and energy. Aim for steady fluid intake throughout the day and include electrolytes—sodium, potassium, magnesium—when you sweat or exercise. Caffeine belongs in the morning hours so sleep can do its job. Alcohol is a saboteur of deep sleep and mitochondrial repair; minimize it and avoid pairing it with late-night eating.

Targeted supplementation fills predictable gaps without relying on brand names. Consider: a methylated B-complex for methylation and energy; concentrated omega-3 (EPA/DHA) for inflammation and brain/joint support; the trio of vitamins A, D3, and K2 (MK-7) for bone, vascular, and hormone receptor health; magnesium (glycinate or threonate at night) for sleep and insulin sensitivity; selenium, zinc, and—in iodine-deficient settings—modest iodine, alongside tyrosine, to support healthy thyroid conversion; diindolylmethane (DIM) to assist estrogen metabolism when symptoms or labs suggest; DHEA in low, lab-guided doses during specific stress seasons; immunoglobulin G concentrates for gut immune support; short-term botanical antimicrobials when overgrowth is documented; and mucosal nutrients such as L-glutamine and zinc carnosine to restore the barrier after insults. These are not forever supplements; they are tools, deployed with testing and reassessment.

Because life is busy, routine beats enthusiasm. Batch-cook proteins and roast vegetables once or twice a week; keep salad greens, olives, nuts, and olive oil ready to assemble; stock quick protein options for chaotic days; and default to a simple template—protein, two vegetables, and an added fat—for most meals. Eat at a table without screens when you can; the act of paying attention reduces how much food it takes to feel satisfied.

Two composite stories show how nutrition unlocks momentum. A 52-year-old woman in menopause with night sweats and joint stiffness builds daily protein to 110–130 grams, adds magnesium at night, and shifts dinner toward vegetables, olive oil, and a measured starch. Estrogen and progesterone support begin; DIM and the A/D/K2 trio are added; within a month sleep steadies and morning stiffness fades. A 58-year-old man with afternoon crashes adopts protein-anchored meals, adds a 10-minute walk after lunch, uses concentrated omega-3, magnesium, and a methylated B-complex, and supports thyroid conversion with selenium and zinc after labs show under-conversion. Four weeks later energy is even; by twelve weeks his waistline shrinks and fasting insulin improves.

Layer this onto BHRT and peptide work with a synergy mindset. Food lowers inflammation and provides raw materials; BHRT restores the messages that tell your body to build and protect; peptides give precision nudges to recovery, tissue repair, and mitochondrial output. People who combine all three—alongside sleep, movement, and stress rhythm—turn progress into a reliable pattern rather than a lucky week.

The goal is not perfection; it is consistency. Choose a default plate you can repeat. Treat meals as messages. When you do, your body responds quickly: sleep firms up, cravings quiet down, training feels purposeful, and labs begin to reflect a younger biology. That is how nutrition adds years to your healthspan—not with a miracle food, but with thousands of aligned choices your cells recognize as safety and possibility.

Chapter 13

Sleep: The Forgotten Pillar of Anti-Aging

Sleep is not time off from life; it is the nightly maintenance window that keeps your biology young. When people finally sleep well, they often describe it the same way: "My body charges overnight again." That feeling is not poetic—it is cellular. While you sleep, hormones synchronize, memories consolidate, synapses are pruned and strengthened, inflammation quiets, the brain's glymphatic system washes away metabolic waste, and mitochondria repair the membranes that make tomorrow's energy. If you want the fastest, most humane way to look and feel biologically younger, start by treating sleep as the pillar that holds up every other pillar. When sleep improves, nutrition choices get easier, training actually sticks, mood evens out, and bioidentical hormone replacement therapy (BHRT) works better because receptors listen. When sleep is chaotic, all of your efforts have to swim upstream.

A good night's sleep is not one thing; it is a sequence. As you drift off, your brain moves from light stages into slow-wave sleep, the deep, high-voltage, low-frequency pattern that children have in abundance and adults lose with age. Slow-wave sleep is where growth hormone pulses are strongest, where tissues repair, and where immune memory is trained. Later in the night, rapid eye movement (REM) sleep surges. REM is metabolically active; it is when the brain stitches emotional tone to the facts you learned, when motor patterns are rehearsed, and when creative problem solving happens in the background. Healthy nights cycle between non-REM and REM four to six times, with more deep sleep early and more REM toward morning. Miss the first third of the night and you miss the most restorative slow-wave sleep; slice off the last third and you lose REM. Either way, you start the day with a deficit you cannot fake your way through for very long.

Hormones do not float above this process; they are choreographed by it. Cortisol follows a circadian rhythm, rising before dawn to prepare you for the day and falling through the evening so you can descend into sleep. When bedtime drifts later and screen light hits your eyes at midnight, that rhythm flattens and you wake at odd hours, restless or wired. Insulin sensitivity is significantly higher in the morning than at night; eating late pushes glucose higher and steals REM as your body juggles digestion instead of deep repair. Leptin and ghrelin, the hormones that govern hunger and satiety, respond to sleep duration and quality; short, fragmented nights elevate appetite and change cravings toward quick energy that doesn't serve you. Thyroid physiology is tied to sleep as well—chronic short sleep alters conversion and can leave you cold, slow, and unmotivated. Estrogen and progesterone shape sleep architecture in women across the lifespan; progesterone has a calming, GABA-supportive effect that eases sleep onset, while adequate estrogen reduces hot flashes and night awakenings and supports REM. Testosterone in men peaks during healthy sleep; when sleep is consistently truncated, testosterone drifts down and training stalls. This is why people say, "Everything works better when I sleep." It is not an opinion; it is the endocrine system behaving the way it is designed.

If you grew up in a culture that glorified hustle and sleep deprivation as a badge of honor, it is worth unlearning. The evidence is clear that chronic sleep loss raises inflammatory markers, impairs insulin signaling, increases blood pressure, and accelerates biological aging signals. Even partial restriction—five to six hours a night for a week—can shift immune gene expression toward a pro-inflammatory state and make your face look older because skin repairs less collagen under the surface. This is not to scare you; it is to give you leverage. If your schedule feels immovable, even a small, consistent increase in sleep time—twenty to thirty minutes more each night—compounds quickly. People who start there report calmer mornings, fewer afternoon crashes, and more capacity to train or cook a healthy dinner. Sleep is a keystone behavior: change it, and other changes become easier.

The relationship between sleep and appetite is one of the most practical examples. After a poor night, people don't crave salmon and broccoli; they crave sugar and starch. That is biology trying to keep you awake. When you fix sleep, cravings decay in force and frequency because ghrelin quiets and leptin speaks up. Likewise, the timing of your last meal has outsized impact. An early, protein-anchored dinner with colorful vegetables gives your body a five-to-six-hour head start on digestion so your heart rate can drift down and REM can expand near dawn. Late dining compresses that window; you will see it on a wearable device as elevated overnight heart rate and less deep and REM sleep. If you do nothing else, pull dinner earlier, dim screens, and give yourself a regular wind-down. Many readers find those three moves deliver disproportionate gains.

The gut and sleep form a loop that either supports you or drags you. Your microbiome produces short-chain fatty acids from fiber and polyphenols that reduce inflammation and talk directly to the nervous system through the vagus nerve. Certain gut microbes influence the serotonin–melatonin pathway; most of your body's serotonin is made in the gut, and melatonin—the hormone of darkness that cues sleep—is synthesized downstream. When the gut lining is irritated by ultra-processed foods, alcohol excess, or dysbiosis, sleep is often lighter and more fragmented. People chalk that up to stress alone, and stress is real, but an inflamed gut whispers into the brain all night long. Repair the lining and rebalance the microbes, and sleep depth often increases even before supplements change. That is why a gut-first reset—eliminating sugar and refined flours, trimming alcohol, favoring whole foods, and using targeted support when needed—shows up so quickly as better sleep on a device and better mornings in your body.

Bioidentical hormone replacement therapy can be a sleep therapy—when it is individualized and monitored. In women, adequately dosed progesterone often shortens sleep latency and reduces middle-of-the-night awakenings by supporting GABAergic calm, while estrogen relieves vasomotor symptoms that steal deep rest. Many women report that the first sign their BHRT dose is right is not daytime energy—it is the first week without 2 a.m. wake-ups. In men, bringing testosterone back to an optimal range helps restore normal sleep architecture by reducing nighttime restless wakefulness and improving next-day vigor, especially when paired with thyroid optimization if conversion has lagged. The goal is not to knock you out; it is to restore normal signaling so the sleep you get is productive. This is also why we tune doses early in a program and then ask you to be boringly consistent. Sleep loves routine; so does hormone signaling.

Peptides and targeted nutraceuticals make a noticeable difference when used to support the fundamentals. If your nervous system is revved from daytime stress, calming daytime support can level the slope so you don't arrive at bedtime with a racing mind. A balanced daytime formula—as many readers know under names like "Calm Day"—helps steady stress responses without sedation so you are not borrowing from tomorrow to survive today. For the evening, a gentle, non-habit-forming sleep blend—think "Sleep Time"—can nudge sleep onset by combining nutrients that support the GABA and serotonin pathways and magnesium to relax muscle and nerve. When chronic stress has flattened your natural cortisol curve, adaptogenic blends such as "AdrenaMax" and restorative evening formulas such as "Adrenal Restore" can help bring rhythm back over weeks. None of these override biology; they cooperate with it. You still need a regular schedule, a darker room, and an earlier dinner. But with those in place, people often say, "I remember what deep sleep feels like."

Occasionally, sleep stalls because of something structural rather than behavioral. If your bed partner reports snoring with pauses, if you wake with a dry mouth and sore throat, or if your blood pressure and weight are climbing despite good habits, ask your clinician about screening for sleep apnea. Untreated obstructive sleep apnea fragments sleep cycles and drives cortisol up; it also raises blood pressure and sabotages hormone optimization. The fix might be as simple as positional therapy and weight loss, or it might include an oral appliance or CPAP. Screening for iron deficiency (by ferritin) is reasonable if you struggle with restless legs; low ferritin is a common, fixable contributor to nighttime agitation. If you are experimenting with evening high-intensity workouts and can't fall asleep, move intensity earlier and keep evenings for gentle walking, mobility, or an easy sauna. The idea is not to be fragile about sleep; it is to remove the few heavy frictions that keep you from the deep cycles your system needs to stay young.

Light is the most powerful environmental cue you control. Morning light anchors your circadian clock, telling your suprachiasmatic nucleus in the hypothalamus that "day has begun"; downstream, cortisol rises appropriately, body temperature nudges up, and metabolism prepares for activity. Twelve to fourteen hours later, the signal to sleep is more likely to arrive on time. Evening light does the opposite. Blue-enriched screen light into the eyes after dusk suppresses melatonin, delays sleep onset, and fragments the first sleep cycle. A simple rule—dim the house and the phone an hour before bed—feels quaint until you try it and notice that sleep comes faster and is thicker. If work or life requires screen use, set devices to warmer tones at sunset and consider blue-light-limiting glasses as backup, not as license to ignore your environment. Darkness is a nutrient; dose it nightly.

Temperature and breathing are underappreciated tools. A cooler bedroom—generally in the mid-60s Fahrenheit for most people—improves sleep onset and maintenance because the body needs to shed heat to fall and stay asleep. A warm bath or shower an hour before bed helps paradoxically by dilating blood vessels at the skin, allowing core heat to dissipate. Gentle breathing practices that elongate the exhale signal the parasympathetic system that it is safe to power down. Three to five minutes of slow, quiet nasal breathing before you turn out the light is not a performance trick; it is a reminder to your physiology that you are not being chased. Many readers keep a journal by the bed and write a "closure script" for tomorrow's top three tasks—this simple act reduces nighttime rumination because your brain doesn't feel responsible for keeping the list active all night.

Caffeine and alcohol deserve a clear framework. Caffeine has a half-life of about five to seven hours in many individuals, longer in slow metabolizers. That means a 2 p.m. coffee can still be half-active after dinner. If sleep is precious, keep caffeine to the morning and use it after you have eaten so you are not propping up low blood sugar with a stimulant. Alcohol is relaxing in the first hour and disruptive for the next several; it fragments sleep, raises heart rate, suppresses REM, and wakes you at 3 a.m. thirsty. If you drink, do so with dinner, keep servings small, and leave several hours before bedtime. Many readers test two weeks alcohol-free and are stunned to discover fewer hot flashes, deeper sleep, and lower overnight heart rate without changing anything else.

The skin and brain are in the sleep story, too. Collagen synthesis, wound healing, and skin barrier repair accelerate at night alongside growth hormone pulses. Chronic sleep loss thins skin and deepens lines because repair windows shrink. Memory and learning likewise depend on sleep; facts move from short-term buffers into long-term storage during deep and REM cycles, and motor skills consolidate. If you want to learn a new lift, a new language, or a new instrument faster, protect your sleep around practice days. If you feel emotionally more volatile after poor nights, that is your amygdala over-reacting without adequate top-down control from the prefrontal cortex—another effect that normalizes when sleep is restored.

For people who like structure, a two-week reset turns this chapter into action. Wake within the same thirty-minute window daily, get outside for light within the first hour, and move your body. Eat a protein-anchored breakfast once morning hunger appears. Cut caffeine by early afternoon. Eat an early dinner built around protein, vegetables, and healthy fat, and make the last bite three to five hours before lights out. Dim screens and house lights an hour before bed; treat this as non-negotiable for the experiment. If stress is high, use a daytime calming formula to smooth the slope and a gentle bedtime blend to ease the transition; if your adrenals are tapped, add restorative adaptogens in the evening. Keep the room cool and dark; use a fan or white-noise if you are noise-sensitive. Walk five to ten minutes after dinner to calm blood sugar. Journal your closure script and practice three minutes of slow nasal breathing. Do it for fourteen nights. You will recognize yourself again.

Where does BHRT fit in the reset? After you have a week or two of predictable sleep timing, review your labs with your clinician. In perimenopause and menopause, consider whether progesterone at night and properly dosed estrogen through the day could remove the two biggest sleep thieves—anxious wakefulness and hot flashes. In men, confirm that low sleep is not artificially depressing testosterone and that apnea is not sabotaging progress; then restore levels methodically. In both sexes, confirm thyroid status and iron/ferritin if fatigue is disproportionate to sleep time. Once sleep is stable, peptide cycles can begin to layer in to target your goals—gut repair to stop nighttime wakings from GI discomfort, mitochondrial support to make mornings brighter, or cognitive blends to ease daytime focus so you are not chasing sleep debt with stimulants. The right sequence is simple: stabilize sleep, normalize hormones, then accelerate with precision tools.

If you worry you have "tried everything," remember that sleep is a system. One or two stuck gears can jam the whole machine. The win is in low-drama adjustments made in the right order. For some, the first change is as prosaic as moving dinner earlier and putting the phone away. For others, it is saying yes to BHRT after years of middle-of-the-night awakenings. For others still, it is replacing an old mattress and pillow that create a pain loop. Progress rarely arrives as a single miracle; it arrives as a collection of ordinary choices repeated nightly.

There is a reason people look different after a month of real sleep. Eyes are clearer because inflammation is down. Skin texture improves because collagen repair is happening on schedule. Training numbers climb because mitochondria are producing energy predictably. Mood stabilizes because the brain is converting experiences into memory rather than letting them rattle your nervous system all night. And there is a quieter, deeper shift that people report when sleep returns: they feel like themselves. The version of you that handles stress with grace, that laughs easier, that chooses better food without a fight—that version is downstream of sleep.

This is the least glamorous and most generous thing you can do for your future. If you build a life where sleep has a rightful place, you will age more slowly not because you hacked anything, but because you cooperated with how humans are built. Let the night do its work. Protect the first third for deep sleep and the last third for REM. Feed your hormones with rhythm. Bring in BHRT when labs and symptoms point that way. Use peptides and nutraceuticals to smooth rough edges without outsourcing the basics. And then watch what happens when your body wakes up charged—not jittery, but ready. That is the feeling you are chasing. It is available. And it begins tonight.

Chapter 14

Stress, Cortisol, and Inflammation

Stress is not a character flaw or a personality type; it is a biology you can measure, train, and heal. For years, people with relentless fatigue, wired-and-tired nights, salt cravings, brain fog, and stubborn belly fat were told their labs were "normal" and their symptoms were "just life." Many of them learned the hard way that what didn't fit a five-minute visit still fit their bodies: a real pattern of dysregulated stress chemistry that traditional language struggled to name. Call it what you like—"adrenal fatigue," HPA-axis dysregulation, maladaptive stress physiology—the lived experience is consistent. The on-switch sticks. The off-switch sputters. And everything that depends on clean on/off signaling—hormones, immunity, mood, digestion, sleep—pays the price. This chapter is your map out of that loop. It explains how the system works, why it breaks, how to test it, and exactly how to rebuild it with food, sleep, movement, targeted nutraceuticals, BHRT when indicated, and peptides that amplify repair. By the end, you will recognize the pattern in yourself or someone you love—and you will know precisely where to start.

Cortisol is the central actor in this drama, but it is not the villain. You need a strong morning surge to get out of bed and meet the day. You need a gentle slope downward through the afternoon so you can think clearly without a jangly edge. You need a low plateau in the evening so sleep arrives on cue. In healthy sleepers, cortisol rises in the last hours of the night—the cortisol awakening response (CAR)—and peaks 30 to 45 minutes after waking before gliding down. You also see small waves of cortisol during the day—ultradian pulses—that fine-tune focus and energy. When the HPA axis (hypothalamus-pituitary-adrenal) is well-tuned, these patterns feel like "presence": you're alert in the morning, steady through the afternoon, and drowsy at night. When the axis is out of tune, the curve warps. You might wake flat and foggy, then get a second wind at 10 p.m. and stare at the ceiling until 2 a.m. You might feel "buzzed but empty," as if your body is pressing the gas and brake at once. You might have normal blood cortisol but still feel "high," because tissue-level cortisol can run hot even when blood snapshots look fine.

Did you know? The adrenal cortex concentrates vitamin C more than many other tissues—your stress machinery literally stockpiles it for steroid hormone and catecholamine synthesis. Under chronic load, vitamin C turnover rises, which is one reason people feel better when they replete it during a rebuild.

The reason you can feel over-amped with "normal" labs is local activation. Inside cells, enzymes called 11β-hydroxysteroid dehydrogenases toggle cortisol's power. 11β-HSD1 activates cortisol from its storage form (cortisone); 11β-HSD2 inactivates it. Visceral fat, chronic inflammation, and sleep loss up-regulate 11β-HSD1 in liver, fat, and brain. Translation: your tissues can be bathing in cortisol's effects even when your bloodstream looks "okay." Meanwhile, DHEA—the quiet counterweight made in the same adrenal layer—can drift low. The cortisol:DHEA ratio tilts toward "go," away from "buffer," and resilience erodes. Restoring that balance is part biology (supply the raw materials, lower inflammation, re-time light, food, and training) and part psychology (teach your nervous system that safety and recovery are available again).

Stress and inflammation are partners. Acute inflammation is the first responder you need to heal a cut or fight a virus. The danger is when that response never flips into the resolution phase—the on-purpose, enzyme-driven clean-up program that shuts off the sirens. Specialized pro-resolving mediators (SPMs), derived from omega-3 fats EPA and DHA, orchestrate that shift. They tell neutrophils to stop swarming, nudge macrophages from attack mode to clean-up mode, and help tissues rebuild without immunosuppression. When sleep is short, food is ultra-processed, and stress is constant, the "start" phase of inflammation works overtime while the "finish" phase stalls. You feel that as puffy joints, morning stiffness, brain fog after illness, allergies that won't quit, or pain that lingers long after the injury should have healed. The fix is not to hammer the system down indefinitely; it's to complete the loop—reduce the sparks and support resolution.

Did you know? Resolution is not "inflammation fading." It is a separate, active program with its own molecules—resolvins, protectins, maresins. That's why people stuck in post-inflammatory funks often feel a gentle, steady lift when they replete omega-3s and, in selected cases, add SPMs: the body finally gets instructions to finish the job.

Zoom out, and the concept that ties this together is allostatic load—the cumulative wear on your systems from repeated adaptation. Your brain triages demands. Your endocrine system changes the fuel mix. Your immune system patrols. Your gut decides what gets in and what must stay out. With intermittent challenges and generous recovery, the team wins. With unending challenges and meager recovery, the team burns out. The results don't require a cytokine panel to recognize: cold hands and feet, a brain that feels one beat behind, a gut that is reactive to everything, skin that flares after stress, workouts that leave you wrecked instead of rebuilt, and moods that flatten or spike. This is the daily face of allostatic load.

Cortisol does not act alone. Thyroid hormones set your base tempo for energy and heat. Under chronic stress, conversion of T4 to T3 slows and more T4 diverts to reverse T3—the brake pedal. Estrogen and progesterone shape stress perception and sleep architecture; when estrogen drops (perimenopause, menopause), joint complaints often rise and sleeping through the night gets harder; when progesterone is low, the brain loses GABA-mediated calm. Testosterone influences drive, muscle repair, and stress tolerance in women and men. DHEA tempers cortisol at immune cells and supports sex steroid balance. When these hormones drift outside optimal ranges, your stress responses become more expensive: more inflammation for the same insult, more fatigue for the same workload, more recovery time for the same workout. Aligning hormones is not "medicating stress"; it is restoring the internal conditions that make resilience possible.

So how do you measure and map this? Start with patterns. A diurnal cortisol test (salivary or dried spot) including the cortisol awakening response shows whether the curve is intact or inverted. DHEA-S tells you if the "brake" is on board. A 24-hour urinary cortisol metabolite panel can hint at how you process cortisol and whether tissue activation is high. Thyroid labs (TSH, free T4, free T3, ± reverse T3) reveal whether stress has put the brakes on metabolism. Inflammation markers like hs-CRP, fibrinogen, and (in complex cases) IL-6 add context. Fasting insulin and a post-meal glucose check expose the blood sugar swings that keep cortisol rescuing you all day. Vitamin D and an Omega-3 Index show whether your membranes and immune system have the raw materials for resolution. Wearables add free daily data—resting heart rate, sleep stages, and heart rate variability (HRV) usually improve in parallel with how you feel when your plan is working.

Nutrition is your first and loudest lever. Anchor meals with complete protein (25–40 grams for most adults per meal), a rainbow of plants, and healthy fats, and put starch to work earlier in the day or around training. This smooths insulin, so cortisol doesn't have to bail you out of sugar crashes. Favor extra virgin olive oil, avocado, nuts, seeds, olives, and fatty fish; use butter or ghee modestly if tolerated. Trim industrial seed oils common in restaurants and packaged foods—they build membranes that are brittle and pro-inflammatory. Add polyphenol-rich spices and foods that calm NF-κB and the NLRP3 inflammasome: turmeric/curcumin, ginger, rosemary, oregano, cocoa, green tea, brightly colored berries, pomegranate. Prioritize omega-3s to elevate your Omega-3 Index; in people stuck in post-inflammatory states, consider adding SPM precursors or concentrates under professional guidance so the "finish" signal is loud enough.

The gut is not just collateral damage in stress; it is a stress organ. Cortisol and adrenaline change motility, lower stomach acid and pancreatic enzyme output, and loosen intestinal tight junctions. That means poorer digestion, nutrient gaps, and immune activation as bacterial components and food fragments slip into circulation. You feel it as bloating, irregularity, skin flare-ups, headaches, and fog. A practical rebuild follows a 5-R sequence: Remove irritants (alcohol excess, ultra-processed foods, fried seed-oil meals; if indicated, short, supervised botanical clears for yeast or parasites). Replace digestive support when needed (bitters, betaine HCl, pancreatic enzymes, bile salts) so food breaks down. Reinoculate with probiotics and, even more importantly, prebiotic fibers from plants. Repair with nutrients like glutamine, zinc carnosine, aloe, and collagen—plus immune-binding IgG to mop up microbial debris. Rebalance with circadian rhythm, movement after meals, and stress practices that keep the vagus nerve engaged.

Now the part most people never get: which ingredients actually move the needle for stress resilience, and why. In the "daytime calm without sedation" lane—the spirit of formulas often labeled "Calm Day"—look for L-theanine (boosts alpha-wave calm and smooth focus), magnesium (glycinate or taurate forms calm NMDA-driven excitability and steady heart rhythm), taurine (supports GABA tone and bile flow), and calming botanicals such as lemon balm or chamomile. You feel these as fewer spikes and easier transitions between tasks. For the "build the stress engine" lane—the spirit of comprehensive daytime adrenal support blends—key micronutrients and adaptogens do the heavy lifting. Vitamin C is a cofactor for steroidogenesis and catecholamine synthesis in the adrenal cortex. Pantothenic acid (B5) builds coenzyme A, the backbone for cortisol, DHEA, and all steroid hormones. Pyridoxal-5-phosphate (active B6) helps you synthesize GABA, serotonin, and dopamine, improving sleep quality and stress patience. Methylcobalamin (B12) and 5-MTHF (folate) support methylation and myelin, stabilizing mood and energy and helping you clear catecholamines cleanly.

Adaptogens—hallmarks of many "AdrenaMax"-style blends—modulate the HPA axis so stress signals are proportionate to the demand. Ashwagandha (standardized for withanolides) has been shown to reduce perceived stress, moderate cortisol, and support thyroid conversion—people feel fewer late-night jolts and better morning energy. Rhodiola (rosavins and salidroside) performs as an anti-fatigue, pro-focus agent, preserving serotonin and dopamine under load—especially useful for brain fog. Eleuthero (eleutherosides) improves endurance and resilience to repeated stressors without jitter. Holy basil (Tulsi) quietly steadies stress reactivity and has friendly effects on glucose and lipids. Schisandra supports hepatic detox balance—practical when stress has overloaded the same liver pathways that process hormones and environmental compounds. Reishi's triterpenes and beta-glucans contribute immune modulation and parasympathetic tone—ideal for evening transitions.

When nighttime cortisol runs high, phosphatidylserine helps by blunting excessive ACTH/cortisol responses, improving sleep depth without next-day fog. Glycine (3 grams) at bedtime can shorten sleep latency and cool the core for deeper sleep. Magnesium again matters here, and in hormonally driven insomnia, oral micronized progesterone (when appropriate and supervised) increases GABAergic calm and reduces awakenings.

Inflammation deserves its own tool kit. Standardized curcumin inhibits NF-κB and COX-2, easing sore joints and "brain on fire" days; bioavailability is key, so look for enhanced delivery forms. Boswellia (AKBA-standardized) balances the 5-LOX pathway—practical for stubborn musculoskeletal aches. Quercetin stabilizes mast cells and can ease histamine-linked anxiety and sleep disruption. Omega-3s improve membrane fluidity and feed SPM production; Vitamin D partners with them for immune balance. N-acetylcysteine plus glycine supplies glutathione precursors, stabilizing redox balance for calmer nerves and deeper sleep. When post-inflammatory fatigue or pain lingers, SPM concentrates can nudge macrophages from attack to clean-up mode, helping you feel like your body is "finishing the story" instead of looping the same chapter.

DHEA belongs in this discussion because it is cortisol's counterweight and a precursor pool for sex hormones. Low DHEA with high or erratic cortisol feels like brittle resilience—things that used to bounce off now stick. Restoring DHEA to optimal, not just "in range," can improve vitality, libido, and stress tolerance in women and men. This is not a DIY supplement; it is a lab-guided tool that you pair with sleep and inflammation work so the benefits stick and excess conversion to androgens or estrogens does not muddy the picture.

Peptides fit naturally once the fundamentals are moving. Selank—a small peptide with anxiolytic properties—modulates GABA-A signaling and dampens pro-inflammatory cytokine chatter; people feel more "quiet clarity" without sedation. Semax increases BDNF expression and antioxidant enzyme activity; under deadline pressure, it helps attention and cognitive stamina. BPC-157, a gastric-derived peptide, up-regulates cytoprotective and angiogenic pathways and supports nitric oxide signaling; in real life, that looks like faster gut and connective-tissue repair so you can train and work without constantly flaring. KPV, an α-MSH fragment, signals through melanocortin-1 receptors to inhibit NF-κB and reduce TNF-α/IL-6—particularly helpful in gut/skin inflammatory loops and post-illness recovery. TB500 (thymosin β-4 analog) supports cell migration and tissue remodeling for stubborn tendon and fascia irritations that keep the stress system "on." MOTS-C, a mitochondrial-derived peptide, activates AMPK and improves metabolic flexibility; users report steadier energy, better glucose handling, and less "crash" in unpredictable schedules. For people whose sleep and recovery need a push, CJC-1295 plus Ipamorelin restore physiologic growth hormone pulsatility; downstream, GH/IGF-1 support connective tissue repair, sleep architecture, and shifting fat away from visceral stores.

Movement is a stress vaccine when dosed sanely. Moderate aerobic work and strength training lower baseline inflammation and raise your stress buffer. Over-training with short sleep does the opposite; it jacks cortisol and inflames tissues. Use a simple heuristic: if you wake unrefreshed with a higher resting heart rate and heavy legs, trade heavy intensity for walking, mobility, or lighter lifting that day. A brisk ten-minute walk after meals trims glucose spikes and signals safety through the vagus nerve. Two strength sessions and two easy cardio days per week, with daily walking, beat sporadic bootcamps by a mile—especially when hormones and sleep are aligned.

Light is the strongest environmental cue you control. Morning outdoor light within an hour of waking anchors your clock: cortisol rises appropriately, body temperature nudges up, and metabolism prepares for daytime tasks. Twelve to fourteen hours later, you are more likely to feel sleepy on time. Evening blue-enriched light suppresses melatonin, delays sleep, and flattens next day's cortisol slope. Dim the house, park the phone, and make darkness a nightly habit you protect like medicine. Temperature helps: a cool room and, paradoxically, a warm shower an hour before bed (which helps shed core heat) make falling asleep easier. Slow breathing with longer exhales (for example, four-count inhale, six- to eight-count exhale) tells the autonomic nervous system it is safe to power down. Two minutes before a high-stakes conversation or presentation can change your day.

Caffeine and alcohol deserve plain language. Caffeine's half-life is five to seven hours for many; slow metabolizers feel it longer. That 2 p.m. coffee can be half-present at bedtime. Keep caffeine in the morning and pair it with food to avoid propping up low blood sugar with a stimulant. Alcohol relaxes you in the first hour and wrecks your sleep for several more—fragmenting REM, raising nighttime heart rate, and spiking next-day cravings. If hormones, sleep, and body composition are priorities, keep alcohol occasional, earlier, and modest during your rebuild.

Did you know? One night of short sleep raises next-day hunger hormones and reduces insulin sensitivity. That's why "willpower" disappears the day after late-night scrolling—you are battling a stack of hormones pushing you toward quick calories.

Safety and nuance matter. Licorice (glycyrrhizin) slows cortisol breakdown via 11β-HSD2 inhibition; it can help specific low-morning patterns but raises blood pressure and lowers potassium in some—use only under monitoring. Some botanicals and amino acids can interact with SSRIs/SNRIs, stimulants, or benzodiazepines—coordinate with your prescriber. Peptides require reputable sourcing and professional guidance. Red flags that call for medical evaluation include unintentional weight loss, darkening skin with salt-wasting, severe dizziness, or suspicion for Cushing's, Addison's, major mood disorders, or sleep apnea. If your bed partner reports snoring with pauses, or you wake with a dry mouth and headache, screen for apnea; untreated, it fragments sleep cycles and drives cortisol up despite perfect habits.

A practical 12-week rebuild ties the science to your calendar. Weeks 1–2: protect sleep ruthlessly—consistent wake time, morning light, early protein-anchored dinner, screens dimmed an hour before bed. Start a daytime-calm blend (theanine, magnesium, gentle adaptogens) and magnesium glycinate at night. Remove alcohol. Begin ten-minute walks after meals. Weeks 3–4: shift food quality—cut ultra-processed snacks, seed-oil fried foods, and late desserts. Add omega-3s and, if lingering post-inflammatory aches persist, consider SPMs temporarily. Begin gut repair: immune-binding IgG, glutamine and zinc carnosine, and, if a clinician advises, a short botanical clear for yeast or parasites. Weeks 5–8: add two strength sessions and two easy cardio days weekly; layer adaptogens (ashwagandha and rhodiola by day; reishi at night). If high cortisol nights persist, add phosphatidylserine at dinner. If aches stall training, consider BPC-157 ± TB500 under supervision. Start MOTS-C if energy and glycemic flexibility limit progress. Weeks 9–12: re-test—diurnal cortisol with CAR, DHEA-S, fasting insulin, Omega-3 Index. Titrate supplements down to the minimum effective stack. Recalibrate BHRT if needed. Keep the sleep/wake anchor, early dinner, and post-meal walks as permanent infrastructure.

Two brief stories bring the pattern to life. A 44-year-old nurse arrived with 2 a.m. wake-ups, afternoon crashes, and weekends lost to recovery. Labs showed a flattened cortisol curve, low DHEA-S, high hs-CRP, and sluggish T3. We rebuilt sleep timing, added theanine-magnesium daytime calm, magnesium glycinate and glycine at night, and a daytime adrenal support blend with vitamin C, B5, B6, and adaptogens (ashwagandha, rhodiola, eleuthero). We ran an eight-week gut repair with IgG and zinc carnosine, added omega-3s plus a short course of SPMs, and brought in MOTS-C for energy. Four weeks later, crashes shrank. Eight weeks later, sleep consolidated. Twelve weeks later, she said, "I feel like my body trusts me again." A 57-year-old architect came in with low drive, joint aches, and weight around the middle despite "eating clean." His CAR was blunted, DHEA-S low, Omega-3 Index poor. We aligned his BHRT, raised protein, cut late alcohol, added omega-3s and Vitamin D, used BPC-157 for elbow/hip pain so he could train, and layered phosphatidylserine at dinner for a month. By three months, his morning energy returned, pain faded, and the scale finally moved.

Did you know? Perceived stress on a questionnaire often tracks with objective metrics: lower HRV, higher resting heart rate, flattened CAR, and slightly higher fasting glucose. When you commit to earlier dinners, dimmer evenings, and morning light for a month, those numbers usually shift with how you feel—proof that behavior is rewriting biology.

The goal is not to avoid stress—impossible and, frankly, undesirable. The goal is to put edges on it and make recovery non-negotiable. Eat like your hormones matter, because they do. Sleep like tomorrow depends on tonight, because it does. Move enough to remind your body it plans to keep its muscle. Use medical-grade nutraceuticals to close gaps quickly: daytime calm for smooth focus; comprehensive adrenal support with vitamin C, pantothenic acid, P-5-P, B12/folate, magnesium, zinc, selenium, phosphatidylserine, and targeted adaptogens; omega-3s and SPMs to lower heat and finish inflammation; DHEA to restore the cortisol balance when labs and symptoms confirm the need. Bring in peptides to accelerate repair where you're stuck. And, when indicated, align BHRT so the same good habits finally pay larger dividends with less friction.

When the on-switch and off-switch work again, ordinary days feel easier and extraordinary days become possible. That is not luck; it is physiology cooperating with your life. Keep going. Your future self is already grateful.

Chapter 15

Brain Health & Cognitive Longevity

Your brain is not a fixed object that slowly dims with time; it is living tissue that remodels itself in response to the inputs you give it. It listens to your hormones, your sleep, your meals, your stress rhythms, your movement, and even your thoughts. When the inputs are right, the brain feels like a clean windshield—clear, bright, and ready. When they're wrong, it feels like fog and friction. The promise of this chapter is simple: most of what people chalk up to "getting older"—the word-finding, the mental fatigue after lunch, the lost thread of a conversation—can be slowed, halted, and often reversed when you align energy, timing, chemistry, and environment.

Start with the big picture. Your brain runs on energy, timing, and chemistry. Energy comes from mitochondria, the little engines inside every neuron and glial cell. Timing comes from sleep architecture and circadian rhythm—the 24-hour clock that coordinates hormone pulses and cellular housekeeping. Chemistry comes from neurotransmitters and the hormones that tune them—estrogen, progesterone, testosterone, thyroid, DHEA, insulin, and cortisol. When energy sputters, timing drifts, and chemistry loses its balance, you don't just feel "off"—you build an environment where cognitive aging accelerates. When you fix them, the brain often surprises you with how quickly it responds.

This is why hormone optimization is a brain story as much as a body story. Estrogen supports synaptic density, blood flow, and glucose utilization in key regions like the hippocampus—your brain's memory librarian. It also modulates serotonin and acetylcholine systems, influencing mood and recall. Progesterone supports GABAergic calm, sharpening your ability to filter noise and fall asleep—one reason thoughtful progesterone support often reduces the 2 a.m. mind-racing that steals the next day's clarity. Testosterone fuels drive, spatial reasoning, and the muscle repair that indirectly protects the brain by keeping insulin sensitivity high. Thyroid hormones set cellular tempo; when conversion from T4 to T3 stalls, brains feel slow even when motivation is strong. DHEA is the quiet buffer that tempers stress chemistry and feeds androgen/estrogen pathways without overstimulation.

The other half of the equation is inflammation. Brains do not like to bathe in inflammatory signals. When microglia—the brain's immune cells—stay "primed," they overreact to small triggers: a short night of sleep, a blood sugar spike, or an argument. You feel it as headachey pressure, irritability, and the sense that concentration keeps slipping out of reach. The solution is not to suppress immunity; it is to shift inflammation into resolution. Omega-3 fats, especially when paired with their downstream mediators (specialized pro-resolving mediators), help the immune system finish its work and leave tissues quieter. You experience that as fewer "brain-on-fire" days and steadier attention.

The gut-brain axis is the third leg of this stool. Your intestines make and metabolize many of the molecules your brain needs to keep mood steady and attention anchored. A balanced microbiome produces short-chain fatty acids that calm inflammation and support the blood–brain barrier. When the gut barrier loosens under stress, poor sleep, alcohol, or processed food, microbial fragments leak into circulation and provoke the immune system. That inflammation doesn't just bother your joints; it blunts mental clarity. A gut reset—remove irritants, replace digestive support when needed, reinoculate beneficial flora, repair the lining, and rebalance habits—often reads in your mind as fewer fog days and easier recall.

Nutrition is the first and loudest way to change the brain's day. Protein-anchored meals keep blood sugar flat enough for stable attention. Colorful plants—especially greens, berries, brassicas, and herbs—bring polyphenols that quench oxidative stress and help your gut microbes make brain-friendly compounds. Healthy fats build flexible cell membranes and feed the production of pro-resolving mediators that finish the inflammatory job. People often notice that when breakfast includes real protein and not just a sweet drink or pastry, their mid-morning feels like a runway instead of a cliff.

Specific nutrients matter because they are the raw materials for your signaling chemistry. Choline donors—citicoline (CDP-choline) or alpha-GPC—support acetylcholine, the neurotransmitter of focus and recall. Phosphatidylserine helps neurons keep membranes supple and can soften stress-induced cortisol spikes that erode memory. B-complex vitamins in methylated forms power the enzymes that build neurotransmitters and clear homocysteine; people feel that as brighter mood and steadier drive. Magnesium, especially glycinate or threonate, stabilizes energy production in mitochondria and helps the nervous system settle at night so memory consolidation can unfold.

Botanicals can play a starring role. Lion's mane mushroom contains families of compounds (hericenones and erinacines) that, in emerging research, encourage nerve growth factor signaling—one reason people often describe "cleaner" recall and calmer mood with consistent use. Bacopa monnieri supports memory consolidation over weeks, not hours—more like compound interest than a jolt. Rhodiola can make heavy cognitive days feel lighter by supporting cellular energy and neurotransmitter balance. Huperzine A is an acetylcholinesterase modulator that keeps acetylcholine active longer—best used in cycles and paired with choline donors rather than as a standalone stimulant.

Sleep itself is where cognitive longevity is minted. Deep sleep—slow-wave sleep—appears to be when the brain offloads trash through the glymphatic system and consolidates key memories. REM sleep connects emotion to memory, defanging the day's stress. When sleep is short or fragmented, attention frays, insulin sensitivity plummets, and your threshold for frustration shrinks. Many people only realize how much sleep was costing them after they fix it: the "background hum" quiets, and thinking feels easy again. Build a consistent wake time, collect morning light, eat dinner earlier, and dim screens an hour before bed. If you need evening support, non-habit-forming blends with magnesium, glycine, theanine, and calming botanicals can smooth the descent without sedation the next day.

Peptides can be powerful when you aim them at the right bottlenecks. Molecules like Selank are used for their calming, anxiolytic profile—supporting GABAergic tone and tamping down inflammatory chatter—so focus feels smooth rather than forced. Semax supports brain-derived neurotrophic factor (BDNF) signaling and antioxidant defenses, which people experience as improved attention, creative flow, and mental endurance on demanding days. NAD+-centered blends paired with BDNF-supportive compounds and choline donors can feel like turning the lights back on when burnout has dulled drive.

In women, brain health pivots across perimenopause and menopause because estrogen's steadying hand on synapses, blood flow, and glucose metabolism begins to drift. This is why women often describe word-finding lapses, patchy sleep, and "I don't feel like me" during this transition. Beyond general nutrition and sleep, specific support can help: cruciferous vegetables and targeted supplements that favor protective estrogen metabolites; omega-3s for membrane health; choline donors and phosphatidylserine to stabilize focus; and, when indicated, bioidentical estrogen and progesterone to restore the signal itself.

Men have their own cognitive pattern as testosterone drifts and visceral fat creeps. Lower testosterone can mean less drive, more indecision, and fuzzier spatial reasoning. Excess aromatase activity in abdominal fat can tilt the balance toward higher estrogens that don't feel good, cognitively or emotionally. The fix is mercifully unglamorous: protein-anchored meals; strength training and walking that lower visceral fat; better sleep; omega-3s; magnesium; and, when indicated, restoration of testosterone and thyroid to optimal—not just "normal"—ranges.

Blood sugar deserves its own paragraph because glucose is both fuel and friction. The brain uses a lot of it, but it wants a steady stream, not a firehose. Spikes followed by crashes feel like sudden irritability, scattered attention, and a hunger that barges into your afternoon and derails your plan. The fix: eat protein and fiber first at meals, push sweets and refined starches to rare occasions, and take a brisk ten-minute walk after larger meals. The difference shows up in your calendar as work that actually gets finished.

Training your brain is training your body. Resistance work three days per week raises BDNF and keeps insulin sensitivity high so your brain runs on stable fuel. Low-intensity movement—a lot of walking—pushes oxygen and nutrients to your brain without the stress spike of all-out intervals every day. Short bouts of cognitive training—learning a language, a piece of music, or a new sport—stimulate plasticity. None of this has to be perfect. It has to be regular. The shape of your week matters more than the heroics of any single day.

The gut repair phase many readers have undertaken for digestion pays cognitive dividends. Immune-binding immunoglobulins mop up irritants in the gut, easing the inflammatory traffic that keeps brains noisy. Targeted botanicals can trim back yeast or parasitic overgrowths that churn out neuroactive metabolites. Nutrients like glutamine and zinc carnosine help restore the gut lining, improving absorption of the very nutrients your brain depends on. When the gut quiets, the brain usually follows. People notice that their fuse lengthens and their recall improves even before the scale or the mirror changes.

If you enjoy understanding "what does what," here is how common brain-supportive ingredients tend to work, stripped of marketing language. Lion's mane brings compounds that up-regulate nerve growth factor pathways and may support myelination; it's a slow, steady builder rather than a same-day stimulant. Phosphatidylserine and phosphatidylcholine provide structural lipids for neuronal membranes and synapses, improving fluidity and receptor function; they also help with cortisol adaptation during stress. Citicoline and alpha-GPC provide choline for acetylcholine synthesis and can support attention without the jagged feel of caffeine. Acetyl-L-carnitine shuttles fatty acids into mitochondria and supports acetylcholine pathways; people often describe clearer morning thinking with regular use. Magnesium threonate may cross the blood–brain barrier more readily than some forms; glycinate calms the body and helps sleep—both show up as better memory consolidation over time. B vitamins in methylated forms (folate as 5-MTHF, B12 as methylcobalamin, B6 as P-5-P) power neurotransmitter synthesis and methylation, lowering homocysteine that can irritate vessels and brain tissue.

A few words about mood, because cognitive longevity is not just about speed; it is about the experience of being you. Chronic low-grade inflammation nudges tryptophan metabolism away from serotonin toward kynurenine byproducts that can aggravate mood. Calming that pathway—through sleep, nutrition, omega-3s, and gut repair—often brightens outlook. Likewise, a drifting cortisol rhythm flattens energy and patience. The fix is circadian hygiene plus tools that smooth stress without sedation during the day: theanine, magnesium, adaptogens such as ashwagandha and rhodiola, and phosphatidylserine at night if cortisol runs high. Pair that with real social connection, light in your eyes each morning, and some time outside where your nervous system can settle.

What about devices and modern habits? Your brain has a budget for attention. Constant notifications shred that budget and leave you feeling "short-wired." Two upgrades make an outsize difference: reclaim mornings as a deep-work zone with the phone in another room, and reclaim evenings as a wind-down zone without blue-enriched light. People often discover that what they thought was "adult ADHD" was their nervous system begging for rhythm and fewer inputs. When they give it that, attention returns to baseline without heroic discipline.

There is room for joy in this plan. Social connection floods the brain with oxytocin and dopamine in ways that heal stress faster than any pill. Natural light, green spaces, and sunlight on your eyes in the morning are free upgrades that anchor your clock and lift mood. Music, novelty, and a sense of progress all tell your brain that life is worth investing in; in turn, the brain invests back with plasticity.

Two short stories make this real. A 47-year-old teacher in perimenopause came in afraid she was losing her edge. Names disappeared, patience ran thin, and sleep broke at 2 a.m. We aligned her sleep timing, rebuilt breakfast with protein and colorful plants, and walked her through a gentle gut reset. We added a brain stack with citicoline, phosphatidylserine, magnesium at night, and lion's mane—all while her clinician dialed in BHRT for estrogen and progesterone. In eight weeks she said, "I feel like my brain is mine again." A 55-year-old entrepreneur who lived on coffee and "catch-up sleep" on weekends rebuilt his week around morning light, early dinners, three strength sessions, and omega-3s. With a NAD+-centered nootropic blend cycled around deep-work days and a choline donor, he described his brain as "quietly fast" instead of frantic.

If you like a simple starting week, try this. Wake at the same time daily and collect ten minutes of outdoor light. Build a protein-anchored breakfast within an hour of waking. Keep caffeine to the first half of the day. Walk after lunch. Do a short resistance session three days per week. Eat dinner three or more hours before bed. Dim lights and screens an hour before sleep. Take magnesium at night. Layer a brain-supportive stack with choline, phosphatidylserine, and lion's mane for eight weeks. If you're working with a clinician and your labs indicate, consider peptide support such as Semax or Selank and align your hormones so the signal gets through.

A word about sources and quality. Many brain-supportive compounds are subtle and cumulative. That means you want consistent, standardized ingredients at doses that match the data and a formula designed to work with your biology rather than against it. The cheapest product is often the most expensive when it doesn't move the needle. Work with trusted clinicians and reputable suppliers, especially for any peptide-based protocol, and pay attention to how you feel at two, four, and eight weeks—not just day one.

Cognitive longevity is not luck. It is the compound interest of a thousand small choices made in the right direction. Feed your brain the materials it needs. Protect your sleep like the high-value appointment it is. Move your body so blood and BDNF keep flowing. Right-size your stress with rhythms that let your nervous system power down each night. Align your hormones so the signal gets through. And, when appropriate, use targeted nutraceuticals and peptides to amplify, not replace, those foundations.

You do not have to accept a smaller life because the calendar turned a page. You can keep your curiosity, your humor, your memory, and your spark. You can feel like yourself at forty, fifty, sixty, and beyond—not by fighting biology, but by cooperating with it. That is the future of brain health, and it is available to you starting today.

Chapter 16

Sexual Health & Intimacy

Sexual health is not a luxury; it is a vital sign. When desire fades, when arousal feels out of reach, when connection turns into logistics, it is easy to assume the relationship is the problem or that "this is what aging looks like." Most couples don't realize that libido, arousal, climax, and intimacy are downstream of biology that can be tuned: hormones that set the signal strength, blood flow that delivers energy, nerves that carry sensation, and a nervous system that knows how to switch from "go" to "rest." When you restore those inputs, intimacy stops feeling like something you have to coax and starts feeling like something your body remembers how to do.

Elena and Marcus didn't come in asking for a miracle. They came in because they were roommates who loved each other and couldn't figure out why they couldn't find each other anymore. She was forty-eight, in the messy middle of perimenopause—waking sweaty at 2 a.m., watching her waistline expand even as she ate "clean," and feeling irritation where curiosity used to be. He was fifty-two, exhausted by mid-afternoon, avoiding intimacy because erections had become unpredictable, and bracing every time she reached for him because he felt like he was letting her down. The old tricks—date night, a weekend away—didn't move the needle, because the problem wasn't romance; it was physiology.

We started where the body listens: with signals and fuel. Their labs told the story many couples carry without a name. Elena's estrogen and progesterone had fallen out of their rhythm, her free testosterone hovered at the very low end of "normal," her thyroid conversion looked sluggish, and inflammatory markers were up. Marcus's total and free testosterone had drifted, estradiol was a bit high for him (common with visceral fat and aromatase activity), and fasting insulin was higher than it should have been. Neither of them had slept through the night in years. We rebuilt sleep timing and light exposure, anchored meals with protein, walked after dinner, and began restoring hormones to optimal ranges—not "average for age," but biologically useful.

Three months later, they were different people—not because they "tried harder," but because their bodies finally had the chemistry that intimacy depends on. Elena's night sweats resolved with properly dosed estradiol; progesterone at night deepened her sleep and quieted the 2 a.m. mind chatter. Low-dose testosterone restored desire and made workouts feel rewarding again. Her brief gut-repair phase eased bloating and steadied her mood. For Marcus, restoring testosterone and trimming visceral fat with protein-anchored meals, strength training, and better sleep improved morning erections and all-day energy. A targeted brain-calm stack during the day (theanine, magnesium, taurine) and omega-3s for vascular health smoothed the edges. They didn't just have more sex; they went dancing again. They hiked. They laughed. Intimacy returned because life returned.

Desire is not a moral quality; it is a network effect. Dopamine and testosterone set curiosity and pursuit; oxytocin and serotonin bring warmth and contentment; estrogen and progesterone tune sensation and a sense of safety; thyroid and cortisol set energy and calm. When cortisol is high and unpredictable, the brain hears "survive," not "connect." When insulin is high and blood sugar wobbles, energy dips steal patience and play. When sex hormones drift or their receptors are muffled by inflammation, the signal doesn't get through. Fix the chemistry and the story changes.

For women, the arousal map often changes with time—and you can change with it. Many are taught that desire should show up first and arousal should follow. During perimenopause and menopause, the order frequently flips: arousal comes first, desire follows once the nervous system feels safe and the body gets the message that connection is welcome. Estrogen maintains vaginal tissue thickness, lubrication, and blood flow; progesterone supports GABA-mediated calm that lets the mind land; testosterone supports spontaneous desire, intensity of orgasm, and pelvic floor tone. As estrogen drifts, the vaginal microbiome changes; the tissue becomes thinner and more easily irritated; lubrication falls. Discomfort becomes avoidance, and avoidance becomes "we're just not that couple anymore." You are not broken. You are under-signaled. Local estrogen—vaginal estradiol or estriol—can restore tissue integrity, pH, and microbiome balance with minimal systemic absorption. Systemic estrogen (in properly dosed, bioidentical form) can re-establish vasodilation and reduce pain, while progesterone at night often ends the 2 a.m. stare-at-the-ceiling that erodes desire. Low-dose, lab-guided testosterone in women is a game changer for many: energy rises, exercise feels rewarding, and mental "spark" returns—desire tends to follow. Thyroid tuning matters too, because a slow thyroid feels like low interest in everything.

Men ride their own chemistry. Erection is a vascular report card—the penile arteries are narrower than coronary arteries, which is why erection difficulties often show up before chest pain. Testosterone supports nitric oxide synthase, dopamine tone, and muscle repair; too little means low drive, more belly fat, and less reliable erections. Excess aromatase activity in abdominal fat converts testosterone to estradiol, which can flatten mood and interfere with function. The fix is mercifully unglamorous: rebuild sleep, eat and train to lower visceral fat, restore testosterone to optimal, and support endothelial health with movement and omega-3s. Many men discover that when they sleep 7–8.5 hours, train consistently, and stop leaning on late-night alcohol, the "mystery" solves itself because blood flow and signaling do.

Did you know? One week of short sleep can drop daytime testosterone in healthy men enough to feel the difference in drive and mood. Fix sleep first and watch how many "libido problems" were really "fatigue problems."

Stress is the hidden third wheel. The body is smart; if it thinks the world is dangerous, it will postpone reproduction. High, erratic cortisol flattens libido in all sexes, narrows attention, and pushes blood sugar to swing. Restoring a clean cortisol rhythm (brisk morning rise, gentle evening fall) often reignites interest because the nervous system can finally power down. Daytime "calm without sedation" support—built from L-theanine (promotes alpha-wave calm), magnesium glycinate or taurate (quiets excitatory NMDA activity), taurine (supports GABA tone), and gentle adaptogens—helps people move through the day without the jagged edges that shut intimacy down by night.

Inflammation silences pleasure chemistry. Chronic inflammatory signaling blunts dopamine, irritates nerves, and tightens blood vessels. Two levers change the tone quickly: nutrition that trims refined sugar and seed-oil-heavy foods, and fatty acids that push the immune system toward resolving the response. Omega-3s (EPA/DHA) incorporate into cell membranes and set the stage for specialized pro-resolving mediators (SPMs)—resolvins, protectins, and maresins—that tell neutrophils to stop swarming, nudge macrophages from attack mode to clean-up mode, and help tissues rebuild. This isn't "anti-inflammatory forever"; it is finish-the-job chemistry that frees your brain from the background alarm.

Blood flow is chemistry plus plumbing. Vasodilation is a nitric oxide story—built from arginine and citrulline and recycled with help from antioxidants. Real food gets you most of the way: beets, arugula, citrus, pomegranate, and cocoa. Consistent movement and strength training increase endothelial nitric oxide synthase, the enzyme that liberates nitric oxide when you need it. Magnesium helps smooth muscle relax; omega-3s keep membranes flexible; polyphenols from berries and dark chocolate help the endothelium behave like young tissue.

Peptides can be potent when they are used to solve the right bottleneck. PT-141 (bremelanotide) stimulates melanocortin receptors in the brain's arousal circuits; it does not change hormones directly, which is why it can be effective across sexes when desire is present but stuck behind anxiety or low signal. Some experience mild nausea; dose, timing, and supervision matter. CJC-1295 paired with Ipamorelin supports physiologic growth hormone pulsatility; downstream, people often notice better body composition, deeper sleep, and more resilient recovery—benefits that indirectly improve desire and performance. BPC-157 and TB500, used under clinical guidance, support connective-tissue and microvascular repair; people feel fewer "hot spots," less post-activity soreness, and more confidence in their bodies.

The O-Shot® and P-Shot®: Platelet-Rich Plasma for Local Repair. Platelet-rich plasma (PRP) concentrates your own growth factors—PDGF, VEGF, TGF-β—and, when injected by trained clinicians into clitoral/vaginal tissues (O-Shot®) or the penile corpora (P-Shot®), aims to improve blood flow, sensitivity, and tissue quality. These specific procedures were developed by Charles Runels, MD, and are offered by certified providers who follow defined protocols. Evidence is evolving and technique matters; think of PRP as a regenerative option that pairs best with systemic work: hormone optimization, sleep, training, and anti-inflammatory nutrition. Many report improved arousal and orgasmic intensity;

importantly, the O-Shot® is also used in programs addressing urinary incontinence for many women. (More information: oshot.info and priapusshot.com/research.)

Tissue quality and sensation matter beyond procedures. Childbirth, pelvic surgery, endometriosis, and simple time can leave micro-injuries in pelvic tissues. A combination of pelvic floor physical therapy and local tissue support changes lives. For women, local estrogen plus targeted repair (often including nutrients like hyaluronic acid and, in some programs, BPC-157 under medical guidance) can reduce dyspareunia and bring confidence back. For men, learning to relax the pelvic floor—not just strengthen it—improves erection quality and reduces premature ejaculation driven by tension.

The gut–sex axis is real. The estrobolome—the collection of gut microbes that metabolize estrogens—shapes estrogen balance; dysbiosis can tilt metabolism toward more reactive estrogen byproducts that irritate tissues. Cortisol and adrenaline change motility, reduce stomach acid and enzyme output, and loosen intestinal tight junctions, allowing microbial fragments to slip into circulation and provoke the immune system. You feel it as bloating, brain fog, skin flares—and a body that doesn't want to be touched. A short "remove and repair" phase—eliminating the usual irritants, binding gut antigens with immunoglobulins, and restoring the lining with nutrients like glutamine and zinc carnosine—often removes surprising friction in the bedroom because it settles the immune system first.

Local ecosystems need care, too. Low estrogen shifts the vaginal microbiome away from protective lactobacilli, increasing pH and irritation. Local estrogen restores the environment; gentle, unscented cleansers, breathable fabrics, and avoiding harsh antimicrobials preserve balance. For men, recurrent penile irritation often tracks with glycemic control and hygiene; lowering sugar and improving insulin sensitivity changes the terrain pathogens love. Simple, boring habits—hydration, gentle cleansing, breathable fabrics—are intimacy tools.

Nutraceuticals can support the entire pathway when they are chosen for what they actually do. A concentrated omega-3 (EPA/DHA) improves endothelial function and provides the raw material for SPMs. Vitamins D3 and K2 (often paired with vitamin A) support immune balance, vascular health, and hormone receptor function. A methylated B-complex powers neurotransmitter synthesis and methylation used for hormone metabolism; people feel it as steadier energy, brighter mood, and less "edge." Minerals matter: magnesium for smooth-muscle relaxation and sleep, zinc for androgen receptor function and nitric oxide support, and selenium for thyroid and antioxidant defenses. Botanicals like saffron, maca, and Panax ginseng have supportive data for mood, arousal, and energy in select groups; they are helpers, not replacements, for the foundations.

Sleep is the bedrock. The best aphrodisiac is a rested nervous system. Magnesium glycinate or taurate in the evening relaxes skeletal and smooth muscle, steadies heart rhythm, and deepens slow-wave sleep. Glycine can shorten sleep latency and improve sleep depth; light discipline—dim house lights and no blue-enriched screens in the last hour—protects melatonin so circadian timing does its work. When sleep normalizes, people are shocked by how quickly desire returns; what they thought was "low libido" was actually "no reserve."

Touch is medicine. Skin-to-skin contact increases oxytocin—the bonding hormone—within minutes and lowers perceived stress. Translation: you do not have to wait for desire to touch; often touch brings desire. Relearning the language of slow, affectionate touch without a goal lowers performance pressure and allows arousal to arrive in its own timing. Many couples rebuild confidence with a weekly "us hour" that has one rule: the point is connection, not completion. Ironically, completion returns when connection returns.

Modern habits deserve honesty. Dopamine is about anticipation, not satisfaction. Endless novelty—from porn to infinite scroll—trains the brain to chase novelty and blunts real-life attraction. Many couples discover that porn-heavy habits shave the edges off connection by over-training the novelty pathway and under-training intimacy. A thirty-day reset—no porn, reclaimed mornings for focus, reclaimed evenings for winding down together—often surprises people with how quickly attraction returns when screens stop stealing the show.

A couple's blueprint makes the science practical. Align sleep first: consistent wake times, morning light, and screens dimmed an hour before bed. Eat protein-anchored meals and walk after dinner. Strength train two or three days per week; add low-intensity walking on non-lifting days. Reduce alcohol to special occasions. Run labs together and review them together; nothing builds connection like working from the same map. Restore hormones to optimal with a clinician who treats symptoms and labs, not labs alone. Add a daytime calm stack if stress keeps hijacking the evening. Bring in targeted peptides or regenerative tools if a clear bottleneck remains after the foundations are solid.

What if desire is still quiet after all this? Check thyroid (free T3), iron status (ferritin in context), B12 and folate, vitamin D, and fasting insulin. Review medications that flatten appetite and libido (some SSRIs, certain antihypertensives, prolactin-raising drugs). Consider psychological safety: are there unresolved resentments, logistical overload, or lack of novelty? Schedule low-pressure experiences that build story and silliness—dancing lessons, a weekend hike, cooking something new together. The brain wants novelty; give it novelty that builds you.

Safety and sanity keep you on the road. Erectile difficulties in midlife can be an early sign of vascular disease—do not ignore them. Check blood pressure, fasting insulin, lipid particle size, and inflammation markers. For peptides and regenerative procedures, work with licensed clinicians who source reliably and screen appropriately (for example, pregnancy, melanoma risk for melanocortin agonists, bleeding disorders for PRP). For hormones, insist on bioidentical forms, individualized dosing, and regular monitoring.

Elena's words say what protocols cannot. "We didn't fall back in love because we bought candles," she told me at their nine-month visit, laughing. "We fell back in love because we had energy again. We went dancing. We hiked. We woke up rested, and by dinner we still liked each other. The sex came back because everything else came back." That is the secret people are rarely told: intimacy is not a standalone project. It is the bonus you get when your brain, hormones, gut, blood vessels, and nervous system agree you are safe and alive.

You deserve a relationship where touch feels like an invitation, not a chore; where desire is not a memory, but a rhythm that returns most days because your life supports it. Optimize the chemistry, rebuild the plumbing, and practice the habits that tell your body, "It's okay to want." Do it together. The payoff is not just better sex. It's a stronger marriage, a happier home, and a body that remembers how to feel alive.

Chapter 17

The Synergy of BHRT, Peptides, and Integrative Medicine

How Smart Sequencing Turns Good Plans Into Great Results

On a Tuesday morning clinic, three people arrived with different stories that led to the same question. A former marathoner in her early fifties, suddenly winded by stairs after a rough year of interrupted sleep and stress, wanted her stamina back. A forty-two-year-old entrepreneur, sharp at work but dimmed at home, wanted to stop swinging between wired and tired. A sixty-one-year-old teacher, cheerful but discouraged by creeping weight and joint stiffness, wanted to feel like herself in her own body. They had each tried to fix things one lever at a time—clean up the diet, push cardio, take a supplement, drink more water, add a sleep app—only to discover what most people eventually learn: when your systems have drifted out of alignment together, single fixes rarely stick. The question was not whether change was possible. The question was in what order to pull the levers so biology would cooperate.

This chapter is about that order. You already know what each pillar can do—how hormones provide the master signals, how peptides nudge stalled pathways back online, how sleep and food set the stage, and how targeted nutraceuticals provide the raw materials that make those signals "land." Synergy is what happens when the pillars stop competing and start cooperating. It isn't a slogan; it's physiology. Hormones tune receptor sensitivity on the surface of your cells, which changes how food feels and how training pays you back. Sleep reorganizes synapses and refuels mitochondria, which makes peptide prompts far more effective. Nutraceuticals provide the cofactors that let all of it translate into real tissue change. When the sequence is right, momentum compounds: better sleep improves insulin sensitivity, steadier insulin improves inflammation, lower inflammation improves hormone signaling, stronger signaling improves training response, and a stronger training response protects sleep. You don't need more willpower when biology starts paying you dividends; you need better timing.

Think of BHRT as restoring the language your body understands. It's not about becoming someone else; it's about regaining the clarity of messages your cells are waiting to hear. When estradiol sits inside its physiologic window, the brain's temperature centers stop overreacting, verbal memory steadies, and joints feel less ancient than your birthdate suggests. When progesterone is present at night, the nervous system exhales, anxiety quiets, and sleep stops fracturing at two in the morning for no reason. When testosterone returns to a healthy female or male range, mornings lean forward again, exercise produces visible returns, and motivation feels internal rather than borrowed. Thyroid completes the orchestra by setting metabolic tempo. An optimized thyroid axis improves mitochondrial biogenesis and helps every other hormone do less work to create the same outcome. BHRT doesn't carry your plan; it allows your plan to carry you.

Peptides act like verbs in that language—short, precise prompts that remind tissues what their day jobs are. Some restore growth-hormone pulsatility so slow-wave sleep deepens and connective tissue finally remodels. Some whisper to mitochondria to improve their efficiency so the same walk burns cleaner and the same workday costs less. Others remind tendons and ligaments that "repair" is still an option after years of micro-injury. A few operate centrally in the brain to lift fog, sharpen focus, and rekindle desire during life stages when those circuits tend to go quiet. None of them replace foundations; they accelerate what foundations are already asking your body to do. Used this way—short cycles, clear targets, clean sourcing—they become multipliers.

Targeted nutraceuticals are the unglamorous heroes. If you ask a cell to build, repair, and signal, it needs materials. Vitamins A, D3, and K2 support receptor literacy, bone mineralization, and vascular integrity so hormone instructions don't bounce. Long-chain omega-3s cool inflammatory noise and protect membranes that carry electrical signals between neurons. Magnesium participates in hundreds of reactions that govern sleep depth, muscle relaxation, insulin behavior, and mood steadiness. Methylated B vitamins keep methylation and neurotransmitter synthesis from becoming bottlenecks when you start living like a higher-output version of yourself. Gut-supporting immunoglobulins and mucosal nutrients reduce the constant immune static caused by a leaky barrier, which is one reason hormone regimens "suddenly" start working when gut work is handled. CoQ10-based mitochondrial support improves electron transport, while dimethylglycine can make oxygen use more efficient in periods of higher demand. These are not random bottles; they are the bolts and beams that let your rebuilding hold.

The smarter question than "What's best?" is "What's first for me?" That's where synergy lives. Start with a clear picture of how your day actually feels, not just the diagnosis code someone once handed you. Does your energy crash in the afternoon? Do evenings feel wired even when you're exhausted? Do you wake before your alarm ready or resentful? Does training feel like a deposit or a withdrawal? Do cravings whisper at night? Is intimacy missing because desire is gone or because energy is gone? Then let labs refine the picture rather than define it: in women, time estradiol and progesterone intelligently if you're still cycling; in both sexes, measure total and free testosterone with SHBG so bioavailability is real, not guessed. Look at DHEA-S for stress resilience, at the full thyroid axis, and at fasting insulin with glucose so you know whether your metabolism is whispering or shouting. Add inflammation markers, vitamin D, ferritin, and a lipoprotein look when possible. If a cortisol curve helps explain why you feel up when you should be down and down when you should be up, get it. You're not collecting trivia. You're mapping leverage.

When sleep is fragmented and stress chemistry is amplified, begin there even if hormones are objectively low. A body that sleeps poorly will fight you on food choices, on training consistency, and on the patience required to adjust doses. Anchor your wake time seven days a week. Step outside into daylight within the first hour even on cloudy days. Keep your bedroom cool and dark, park screens elsewhere, and move stimulants earlier. If a cycling or perimenopausal woman's progesterone has quietly faded, bedtime micronized progesterone often restores continuity quickly—one of the few "fast wins" in physiology. If growth-hormone signaling is clearly blunted by years of sleep loss, a brief course of a gentle secretagogue stack can deepen slow-wave sleep enough that everything else becomes easier. Then, and only then, judge food, training, and hormones. You will make fewer mistakes when you obey biology's order of operations.

When fatigue and slow recovery headline your week, create a floor you can stand on before you complicate your stack. Eat enough protein to support repair—roughly 1.6 to 2.0 grams per kilogram of body weight per day for active adults—and distribute it across meals. Lift twice or three times a week with compound movements and progressive overload scaled to your actual life. Walk daily. Then evaluate hormones and mitochondrial support. It is astonishing how often a "hormone problem" reveals itself as an input problem when consistency returns—just as it is astonishing how often truly low hormones reveal themselves as the reason consistency could never stick. If composition is stuck, especially visceral fat through midlife, look beyond calories. Begin with protein-anchored meals, move for ten minutes after you eat, scale two interval sessions a week to your current capacity, push alcohol earlier and rarer, and then correct suboptimal hormones so your body stops acting like you are still in energy conservation mode. Thyroid conversion and estradiol/testosterone balance don't replace discipline; they make discipline fair.

Safety is part of synergy. Optimizing estradiol, progesterone, testosterone, or thyroid is thoughtful, individualized work. The right dose lives in physiology, not in bravado. The aim is to restore function without drifting into signals that tell you the dose is ahead of the plan: breast tenderness that persists past the adjustment period, fluid retention that doesn't settle, oily skin or chin hair in women, blood pressure or hematocrit trending too high in men, or a jittery, overcaffeinated feel on thyroid. You don't abandon a helpful hormone because a dial needed a nudge; you adjust the dial and watch the pattern. In the same way, peptides should be sourced responsibly and run in cycles with clear goals and off-ramps, not treated as forever-pills. Nutraceuticals do their best work when the brand is transparent and third-party tested, when forms are bioavailable, and when you're willing to take them consistently enough for biology to notice.

Adaptation is the point. You won't be in the same season six months from now, and neither should your plan. In early perimenopause, a woman may need nervous-system support at night and a steady supply of progesterone while ovulation fades in and out. Months later, as estradiol drops and symptoms migrate from mood and sleep to joints and thermoregulation, a stable, non-oral estradiol route will often do more than a thousand hacks. A tiny female dose of testosterone can make training pay off again and help desire return as a spark rather than a task. A man who starts with objectively low testosterone might first feel the world sharpen; as he trains consistently and trims central fat, the needed dose often falls because his own receptors have become better listeners. People recovering from head injury or years of shift work often present with flattened growth-hormone rhythms; for them, sleep-focused peptide cycles early in the plan make BHRT feel like it should. Surgical menopause is its own category. When the ovaries are removed or shut down by treatment, the body does not get time to adapt. In that case, earlier support is kinder and safer. Restore estradiol and progesterone appropriately, consider a physiologic dose of testosterone for muscle and desire, and prioritize sleep-protective routines while the nervous system finds a new baseline.

Travel and high-stress seasons are where many plans die, so build what I call a red-zone protocol before you need it. Choose two non-negotiables and stage them everywhere: a magnesium that loves your gut and an omega-3 you tolerate. Keep protein you genuinely like in your bag so airport kiosks don't decide your week. Anchor wake time and light exposure wherever you land, walk after the biggest meal, keep alcohol tiny, and eat the earlier dinner your circadian rhythm will thank you for. If you're on hormones, mind your refill timing so trips don't become dose gaps. If peptides are part of your plan, favor sleep-supportive and repair-support cycles around travel rather than performance ones. Drop the perfectionism. Keep the floor.

Support should respect real budgets. A "good" tier that moves almost anyone forward includes honest sleep hygiene, protein-anchored meals, two or three resistance sessions a week, daylight walks, magnesium in the evening, omega-3s with your first meal, and a methylated B complex for energy and mood. A "better" tier adds individualized BHRT when symptoms and labs agree, plus a small number of targeted formulas that fit your pattern—vitamins A/D/K2 for receptor literacy and bone, immunoglobulins for a noisy gut, and CoQ10 for a tired engine. A "best" tier layers in short, precise peptide cycles for sleep, repair, mitochondrial efficiency, or central focus when foundations are steady. The goal isn't to collect tools. It's to carry exactly what your season requires and nothing you won't use.

Monitoring should be as humane as it is precise. Numbers matter, but so does how life feels on a Tuesday afternoon. Early on, repeat labs every twelve to sixteen weeks to confirm you're in physiologic windows and to catch the rare outlier. As you stabilize, widen the interval. Pair data with a short weekly check-in that asks the same questions every Sunday: Did you sleep through the night? Did you wake ready? Did you think clearly mid-day? Did you recover from training or long workdays? Did stress feel like a solvable problem or an existential threat? Did connection and desire show up? When those curves rise together, keep going. When one drops, don't invent drama; look for the simplest missed lever—often sleep drift, protein slippage, lost walks, or an overdue dose adjustment.

Biology happens in a household, so a brief word about partners and families. When couples optimize together, the plan gets lighter. Sleep schedules line up, kitchens get stocked with the same staples, evening walks become minutes together rather than chores, and intimacy returns as a daily kindness rather than a scheduled task. Parents who reclaim energy and patience create a climate their kids can feel; the model of adults who lift, sleep, cook, and measure what matters is a gift no lecture can match. And if one partner goes first, invite the other with curiosity rather than conversion. Results are persuasive.

So what happened to those three people from Tuesday? For the former marathoner who feared her engine was gone, sleep came first. Bedtime progesterone and a short sleep-deepening cycle turned her nights from fragments to continuous stages. Two weeks later, we added transdermal estradiol for joints and cognition, and a physiologic female dose of testosterone when training still felt flat. As energy returned, she ran scaled intervals twice a week, lifted twice a week, ate protein at breakfast, and added CoQ10 to support the engine. For the entrepreneur stuck between wired and tired, we addressed the cortisol rhythm with daylight and meals on a clock, restored testosterone from "low-normal" to optimal, used a mitochondrial-supportive stack on work sprints, and layered a repair peptide around his shoulder that had quietly edited his training for years. By month three, he described his days as "quietly energized" instead of up-and-down. For the sixty-one-year-old teacher, we began with gut repair so nutrients stopped bouncing off an irritated barrier, added A/D/K2 and omega-3s for bone, brain, and joints, brought estradiol and progesterone back to physiologic ranges, and used tiny doses of testosterone for muscle and motivation. She didn't train like a twenty-year-old; she trained like a strong sixty-one-year-old and watched her stairs stop negotiating with her knees.

If there's one lesson to carry from this chapter, it's that your body is not waiting for perfect conditions to improve. It is waiting for aligned ones. Restore the language of your hormones so your cells know what you're asking. Use peptides like punctuation, not paragraphs—well-timed, clear, and brief. Feed your body materials worthy of the structures you want it to rebuild. Protect sleep like it protects you. Lift something heavy, walk after you eat, and step into the daylight that tells your clock what time it is. Keep your plan personal, data-informed, and seasonally adjusted. That is integrative medicine as it should be practiced: not a bag of hacks, but a coherent method that brings your systems back into conversation. When the conversation is clear, the work feels lighter and the results feel inevitable. Turn the right dials, in the right order, for long enough—and you will look back and barely recognize the version of you who thought decline was the default.

Chapter 18

Cardiometabolic Health & Vascular Longevity

Cardiometabolic health is the quiet headline of aging. Long before a diagnosis appears in a chart, your biology is sending notes: a little more puffiness after meals, blood pressure that creeps, brain fog on a hard afternoon, workouts that feel heavier than they should. These are not random annoyances; they are signals from your heart, blood vessels, liver, pancreas, and muscles that the system is leaning toward "store and protect" instead of "burn and rebuild." In practical terms, this means insulin sensitivity is slipping, endothelial cells are making less nitric oxide, and inflammation is whispering just loudly enough to change how you feel most days. The good news is that these are not fixed states. With the right sequence—optimize hormones, repair the gut, train your muscles, sleep like it matters, and feed your mitochondria—you can make arteries feel younger and metabolism more responsive, often within weeks.

This is not a theory chapter. It is a map. You will see how estrogen, progesterone, testosterone, thyroid, and DHEA orchestrate fat distribution, glucose control, vascular tone, and lipid handling. You will understand why visceral fat is inflammatory and why it behaves differently than the fat under your skin. You will learn how nitric oxide (NO) is created, why endothelial cells stop making enough of it under stress, and what to do nutritionally and therapeutically to restore it. You will see why sleep deprivation pushes blood pressure up and insulin sensitivity down, and how a simple walk after meals can change post-prandial glucose enough to reduce endothelial "friction." Layer in peptides that support tissue repair and mitochondrial output, and nutraceuticals that provide the exact cofactors for vascular resilience, and cardiometabolic "aging" becomes a reversible pattern instead of a fate.

Hormones are the cardiometabolic conductors. Estrogen enhances insulin sensitivity in muscle and liver, protects endothelial nitric oxide synthase (eNOS), and supports healthy HDL function. When estrogen drops in perimenopause and menopause, blood pressure tends to rise, LDL particle quality can worsen, visceral fat accumulates, and the endothelium becomes less responsive. Progesterone calms the sympathetic nervous system and helps with sleep architecture; better sleep, in turn, improves insulin sensitivity and morning blood pressure. Testosterone supports muscle protein synthesis, endothelial function, and fat distribution in women and men; too little means less muscle and more visceral fat, which worsens insulin resistance. Thyroid hormones set the tempo of every cell; when conversion to free T3 lags, resting energy output sinks, LDL rises, and "water weight" hangs around. DHEA quietly buffers cortisol, supports immune balance, and feeds downstream sex hormones; low DHEA with jittery cortisol often shows up as stubborn belly fat and afternoon crashes.

Insulin resistance is not a character flaw; it is a traffic problem. In a healthy cell, insulin knocks and the door opens—glucose enters, mitochondria turn it into ATP, and the system hums. In early insulin resistance, the door gets sticky. Muscles do not take up glucose efficiently after meals, the liver keeps making glucose at the wrong times, and the pancreas compensates by sending louder insulin signals. Over time, high insulin pushes fat storage, especially in the liver and around the abdomen, and high glucose caramelizes proteins (glycation) that stiffen vessels and cloud thinking. Optimizing hormones changes the traffic lights—testosterone and estradiol improve GLUT-4 activity in muscle, progesterone improves sleep so cortisol can normalize, and thyroid tuning restores basal metabolic rhythm. Training acts like a detour—contracting muscle pulls in glucose even when insulin signaling is sluggish. Nutrition clears the road—protein-anchored meals with fiber and low-glycemic plants keep post-meal spikes small enough that the pancreas can whisper again.

Vascular aging is largely an endothelial story. Your endothelium—a single layer of cells lining every blood vessel—creates nitric oxide to tell the smooth muscle in the vessel wall when to relax. Shear stress from healthy blood flow, sunlight, polyphenols, and regular movement upregulate eNOS. Inactivity, hyperglycemia, high triglycerides, smoking, sleep loss, and chronic stress downregulate eNOS and oxidize NO before it can do its job. As NO fades, vessels stiffen, blood pressure rises, and organs see fewer nutrients with more "wind shear." Restoring NO biology requires both signaling (give eNOS the nudge to work) and substrates (give it the building blocks to make NO) while protecting the product from oxidative loss.

Circulation is chemistry plus building blocks. A formula like CircuCORE pulls together the parts your endothelium uses to generate and protect nitric oxide while supporting the matrix around your blood vessels. Vitamin C provides antioxidant support and is a cofactor for collagen synthesis, which strengthens vascular walls. Methylated folate (as Quatrefolic®) helps convert homocysteine to methionine; keeping homocysteine in check protects the endothelium and supports NO bioavailability. Beet root supplies dietary nitrates that your oral microbiome can reduce to nitrite and then to NO, a parallel pathway that complements eNOS. L-citrulline and L-arginine provide substrate for NO synthase; citrulline is often the superior oral source because it bypasses first-pass metabolism and is later converted to arginine in the kidneys. ActiVin® grape seed extract (rich in oligomeric proanthocyanidins) protects NO by reducing oxidative stress and helps maintain healthy capillary permeability. Hawthorn supports coronary blood flow and gentle inotropy. Together, these ingredients create a biochemical environment where vessels can relax when asked and remain resilient under daily stress.

Lipids matter, but context matters more. Total cholesterol alone is an unreliable compass. Apolipoprotein B (ApoB), LDL particle number, triglycerides, HDL function, and the triglyceride-to-HDL ratio tell a clearer story of risk. Hormones influence this map: estrogen tends to improve LDL receptor activity and HDL dynamics; low thyroid inflates LDL; low testosterone raises triglycerides and erodes HDL. Nutrition pushes in both directions depending on quality. Ultra-processed foods and seed-oil-heavy diets oxidize lipids and stiffen membranes; olive oil, nuts, avocado, and fatty fish build flexible membranes and improve receptor behavior. Strength training reduces triglycerides by increasing muscle's capacity to clear and burn fat; zone-2 aerobic work raises mitochondrial density so your heart and skeletal muscle prefer fat for fuel at rest and during easy movement.

Calcium belongs in bones, not arteries. Vitamins A, D3, and K2 work as a team to make that happen. ADK10 supplies these in forms your body likes: vitamin A supports epithelial integrity and gene expression; vitamin D3 improves insulin sensitivity and immune rhythm; vitamin K2 activates matrix Gla protein and osteocalcin, guiding calcium into bone and keeping it out of soft tissues. In a person with suboptimal D and K intake, calcium can drift where it doesn't belong—tightening vessels and stiffening the pulse. Pairing ADK10 with a protein-anchored diet and resistance training strengthens bone while keeping arteries supple.

Mitochondria sit at the crossroads of energy and vascular tone. When the electron transport chain is sluggish, cells struggle to make ATP, and anything that requires energy—ion pumps that regulate blood pressure, the heart's contraction, brain focus—feels harder. Coenzyme Q10 is an essential electron carrier in that chain, shuttling electrons from complexes I and II to complex III. It also stabilizes membranes and acts as an antioxidant. EnerCoQ10 provides a meaningful dose of CoQ10 in a chewable wafer, often helpful for people on statins (which deplete CoQ10) or anyone with fatigue and muscle heaviness. People often describe smoother energy, better exercise tolerance, and calmer heart rhythm after two to four weeks.

DMG deserves its own paragraph. N,N-dimethylglycine functions as an indirect methyl donor and a metabolic buffer. It supports the synthesis of neurotransmitters, nucleic acids, and immunoglobulins, and it improves oxygen utilization at the tissue level. In practice, EnerDMG is used to smooth the physiologic stress of training blocks, long workdays, altitude, and immune challenges. People feel it as steadier endurance, cleaner recovery, and, for many, better concentration without stimulation. On the cardiometabolic front, DMG's support for methylation helps maintain healthy homocysteine, while its effect on cellular respiration complements CoQ10 in the mitochondria.

Blood pressure is a rhythm problem as much as a plumbing problem. The healthiest blood pressure pattern rises briskly in the morning and falls gently in the evening. Magnesium is foundational here: it helps vascular smooth muscle relax, modulates calcium channels, and calms excitatory neurotransmission. A comprehensive formula like Mag Complete that includes well-absorbed forms—glycinate, malate, and taurate—covers muscle relaxation, mitochondrial energy support, and heart rhythm stability. Taurine itself supports bile acid formation (useful for lipid handling) and GABA tone (useful for easing sympathetic overdrive). When magnesium and taurine are in place and sleep is consistent, many people watch their evening blood pressure drift down without changing anything else.

Homocysteine is an under-appreciated signal. Elevated homocysteine irritates the endothelium, impairs nitric oxide signaling, and increases oxidative stress. Methylated B vitamins—folate as 5-MTHF, B6 as P-5-P, and B12 as methylcobalamin—convert homocysteine to methionine and cysteine, reducing vascular friction. Super B, a methylated B-complex, provides those active forms along with riboflavin and niacin to support the enzymes of mitochondrial energy production. People often notice the difference as brighter energy and smoother mood in the first few weeks; labs typically show homocysteine trending down over one to two months when paired with protein-forward nutrition.

Glycemia leaves fingerprints everywhere. Hemoglobin A1c shows average glucose exposure; fasting insulin shows how loud the pancreas is shouting to keep glucose normal; post-meal glucose tells you how the system behaves in real life. You want all three. If A1c is drifting up while fasting insulin climbs, you are storing fat in the wrong places. If post-meal glucose is spiking and lingering, your muscles need more stimulus and your meals need more protein and fiber. BHRT increases the reward for doing the right things by restoring muscle-building signals and improving sleep; training provides the demand signal that tells the body to put glucose to work; nutrition keeps the peaks gentle so recovery can happen.

Inflammation is supposed to turn on, solve a problem, and turn off. When it turns on and never quite turns off, you get a little stiffer each week, a little foggier each month, and your blood vessels act older than your birth certificate says. Omega-3s push the immune system toward resolution. Specialized pro-resolving mediators (SPMs)—made from EPA and DHA—are the "cease-fire" signals that tell neutrophils to stop swarming and macrophages to clean up calmly. A high-quality omega-3 concentrate is step one; SPM-rich concentrates can be layered in for stubborn, smoldering cases where joints, gums, or labs (like hs-CRP) keep telling you the fire never really went out.

The gut–liver–vascular axis is real. Endotoxins such as lipopolysaccharide (LPS) slipping through a porous gut wall are potent triggers of insulin resistance and endothelial irritation. If your belly is bloated by evening, your skin flares unpredictably, and you feel achy after certain meals, your gut is asking for attention—and your arteries are listening. A short, focused "remove and repair" phase can change the terrain quickly. Remove common irritants and ultra-processed foods. Bind and neutralize microbial fragments with GI complete and immunoglobulins (IgG). Repair the lining with glutamine and zinc carnosine. Re-introduce fiber and polyphenols to feed the species that help metabolize estrogen and bile acids properly. Many people feel the shift in two to four weeks: flatter belly, steadier energy, calmer skin, and better sleep—exactly the signals that blood pressure and glucose like to follow.

Did you know that erectile difficulties in midlife often precede a cardiovascular diagnosis by years? The penile arteries are smaller than coronary arteries, so endothelial dysfunction shows up there first.

Rather than reaching only for short-acting band-aids, take it as the nudge to rebuild NO production, improve insulin sensitivity, reduce visceral fat, and restore sleep. The same plan that helps the bedroom is the plan that helps your heart and brain.

Training is medicine for arteries. Resistance training increases muscle mass—the single most important glucose sink you can build—while zone-2 aerobic work raises mitochondrial density and lactate clearance. Short walks after meals are a powerful, overlooked tool: ten minutes can blunt a glucose spike enough to reduce oxidative stress and endothelial friction. In people returning to training after years away, peptides like BPC-157 and TB500 can support tendon and fascia repair so the plan is sustainable, while CJC-1295/Ipamorelin helps recovery and sleep so routine becomes consistency, and consistency becomes results.

Women deserve a special note here. Cardiovascular risk accelerates after menopause not because women "fall apart," but because estrogen's protective effects on the endothelium, lipids, and insulin sensitivity fade. Restoring estradiol in bioidentical form—alongside progesterone and appropriate low-dose testosterone—does more than cool flashes. It normalizes vascular tone, improves sleep, preserves muscle, and reduces visceral fat. Those changes echo as lower blood pressure, better lipid particle quality, steadier glucose, and higher energy to train—four levers that move risk in the right direction.

Men benefit just as clearly. Optimizing testosterone within a healthy range improves insulin sensitivity, reduces visceral fat, and supports endothelial function, especially when body composition and sleep are addressed simultaneously. Men with higher aromatase activity in visceral fat often feel flat because more of their testosterone is converting to estradiol; strength training, lower nightly alcohol, better sleep, and omega-3 intake reduce that pressure. When needed, DIM Plus supports favorable estrogen metabolism as body composition improves.

Blood sugar, lipids, and blood pressure do not improve in isolation; they improve together when the right levers are pulled. A practical plan looks like this in real life without breaking into bullet points. Wake at a consistent time and get morning light in your eyes to set your clock; that single habit lowers nighttime cortisol and steadies blood pressure. Eat a protein-anchored breakfast, saving ultra-starchy foods for days with hard training. Take a brief walk after meals. Place a strength session on your calendar two to three times per week, with one to two sessions of easy aerobic work. Build dinner around protein and vegetables and finish eating two to three hours before bed. Use Mag Complete in the evening, Super B in the morning, Super Omega 3D daily, and ADK10 with meals. Add CircuCORE when blood pressure, cold hands/feet, or endurance hint that your vessels want more NO support. Consider EnerCoQ10 if energy or statin use point to mitochondrial help; add EnerDMG when long days, altitude, or heavy training blocks stretch your recovery bandwidth.

Homocysteine, ferritin, and fasting insulin are inexpensive labs that punch above their weight. Keep fasting insulin in the low single digits, ferritin in context with iron saturation and inflammation markers, and homocysteine in the normal-low range with methylated B support. Check ApoB and, if family history or other risks suggest it, lipoprotein(a). If blood pressure is consistently high despite lifestyle work, check for sleep apnea and check your evening routine; the last two hours of the day decide what your vessels will be asked to tolerate overnight.

Big picture, cardiometabolic rejuvenation is not about perfection; it is about momentum. When you stack the signals in your favor—hormones that say "build and repair," peptides that unlock bottlenecks, nutrition that calms the immune system, and nutraceuticals that supply the exact cofactors for vascular and mitochondrial youth—the body changes back. Blood pressure softens. Post-meal energy stays smooth. Workouts give more than they take. Hands and feet feel warm. Mood steadies. Brain fog lifts. Libido returns. Labs follow life—because you changed the inputs.

If you have felt stuck in the "gray zone" of almost-healthy—labs that are "fine," but a life that feels like a slow leak—this is your exit ramp. Rebuild sleep. Eat like your arteries are listening. Pick up weight and teach your muscle to burn sugar again. Optimize hormones so the effort pays off. Use targeted nutraceuticals to give your endothelium, mitochondria, and nervous system what they need: CircuCORE for nitric oxide and vessel tone; Super Omega 3D and SPMs for inflammation resolution; ADK10 for calcium direction and receptor function; Super B for methylation and energy; Mag Complete for vascular relaxation and sleep; EnerCoQ10 and EnerDMG for mitochondrial output and oxygen use. Add peptides to solve bottlenecks and keep going until ordinary days feel easier and extraordinary days become possible again.

Chapter 19

Skin, Hair & Aesthetic Longevity

Your skin and hair are not vanity projects. They are status reports from your biology—daily readouts of hormones, nutrients, circulation, inflammation, and the way you sleep, eat, and handle stress. When your face looks dull, when acne flares, when your scalp sheds more than it used to, when fine lines seem to deepen overnight, your body isn't betraying you; it's speaking to you. The message is simple: repair is lagging behind wear. The fix isn't a single serum. The fix is to change the environment those cells live in so that repair can outpace wear again.

This chapter stays strictly with the levers you control from the inside and at the surface: food choices that quiet inflammation; hormone optimization that protects collagen and circulation; gut repair that halts immune irritation; nutraceuticals that deliver exact building blocks; peptides that nudge targeted healing; and clean topical routines that support the biology you're rebuilding. No injections or devices here—just a blueprint for making skin and hair look like you actually feel when your system runs well.

Start with what skin and hair actually are. Skin is an immune organ, a vascular organ, a nervous organ, and a barrier—four million square millimeters of intelligent fabric. The epidermis turns over roughly every month, but the deeper dermis turns over much more slowly, which is why collagen loss shows up as sag and laxity over years. Hair is a cycle—anagen (growth), catagen (transition), and telogen (rest)—and each follicle runs its own clock, coordinated by hormones, nutrients, microcirculation, and local inflammation. When systems fall out of sync, more follicles slip into rest and shedding accelerates. When you restore the inputs, the cycle lengthens again.

Hormones write much of the story in the skin and scalp. Estrogen helps keratinocytes and fibroblasts communicate, maintains water content in the dermis, and protects blood flow by supporting nitric-oxide production. As estrogen declines in perimenopause and menopause, the dermis thins, transepidermal water loss increases, and fine lines become more visible—not because you suddenly aged, but because the signal to maintain collagen has faded. Progesterone brings a different gift: a calmer nervous system via GABA pathways and better sleep architecture. Deeper sleep, in turn, raises growth hormone pulses that drive nightly skin repair. Testosterone supports protein synthesis in both sexes and helps maintain the jawline and muscle tone that frames the face; out of range, it can either flatten energy (too low) or worsen oil and acne (too high relative to estrogen). Thyroid hormones are the tempo—when free T3 is low or conversion is sluggish, skin dries, hair gets brittle, and shedding increases. DHEA is a quiet buffer that supports moisture, immune balance, and downstream sex hormones.

Inflammation and insulin are the hidden sculptors. High glycemic swings glycate collagen (think: sugar crust on crème brûlée) and stiffen what should be supple. Ultra-processed seed-oil-heavy diets feed inflammatory eicosanoids that make acne angrier, rosacea redder, and fine lines deeper by degrading collagen with matrix metalloproteinases. Calm the swings, change the oils, and you change the texture. That is why the simplest cosmetic move many people ever make is a food shift: protein-anchored meals, colorful plants, and healthy fats with very few packaged foods. Within weeks, people often notice less puffiness, calmer breakouts, and a glow that makeup can't fake.

The gut–skin axis is the keystone. A porous gut leaks microbial fragments like lipopolysaccharide (LPS) into circulation; your immune system hears "danger" and inflames everywhere tissues are thin and richly innervated—like the face. Dysbiosis also alters estrogen metabolism in the estrobolome, tilting some women toward estrogen-dominant acne or melasma, and some men toward dull, inflamed skin. The repair sequence is simple and powerful: remove irritants, bind and neutralize what shouldn't be there, and rebuild the lining. IgG concentrates bind microbial antigens and toxins in the lumen so they can be carried out; Remove Complete supports short, focused cleanses by supplying botanicals that discourage overgrowth while sparing beneficial flora; ParaKill and CandiKill target parasite and candida burdens when history and symptoms suggest they are part of the problem; and GI Complete provides glutamine, zinc-L-carnosine, soothing demulcents, and immune-balancing nutrients to knit the barrier back together. Within a month, many notice less bloat by evening, fewer breakouts after meals, and steadier mood—the same immune irritation that shows on your face fogs your brain.

Collagen is not a miracle powder; it's a construction project. Fibroblasts build collagen from amino acids—glycine, proline, lysine—with vitamin C as an essential cofactor for hydroxylation and cross-linking. They also need copper and silica to stabilize the matrix. This is why a high-quality diet plus targeted support changes the dermal "bounce." Protein first at meals, bone broth or collagen peptides if intake is low, vitamin C daily, and mineral sufficiency (including copper in balance with zinc, and bioavailable silica) give the skin raw materials to rebuild. Vitamin A in its bioactive forms (from diet or ADK10) supports epidermal differentiation and collagen signaling; vitamin D3 and K2 in ADK10 support immune balance and direct calcium away from soft tissues, preserving vascular flexibility that skin depends on for nutrition.

Circulation is the lifeline for skin and hair. If the microvessels feeding the dermis and scalp are stiff or constricted, even perfect nutrition can't arrive in time. CircuCORE brings the chemistry the endothelium uses to make and preserve nitric oxide: vitamin C to protect the signal and support collagen in vessel walls; methylated folate (Quatrefolic®) to recycle homocysteine and ease endothelial friction; beet root to provide nitrates that convert to nitric oxide; L-citrulline and L-arginine as substrate for nitric-oxide synthase with citrulline improving arginine bioavailability; and polyphenols such as grape-seed oligomeric proanthocyanidins and hawthorn to protect the endothelium from oxidative stress while gently improving perfusion. People often describe warmer hands and feet, faster post-exercise flush, and, over weeks, a healthier scalp "feel"—that is microcirculation waking up.

Mitochondria are the quiet power in beauty. Every centimeter of skin and each hair follicle is loaded with mitochondria that pay the energy bill for repair. When that electron transport chain slows, repair lags and the surface tells on the inside. EnerCoQ10 delivers coenzyme Q10—an electron shuttle and membrane stabilizer—alongside supportive antioxidants to help the heart and skin make ATP. EnerDMG supplies N,N-dimethylglycine, an indirect methyl donor and metabolic buffer that improves oxygen use under stress, whether that stress is a hard workout, a long flight, or a season of poor sleep. In people who feel like their skin looks "tired" by afternoon, supporting mitochondrial throughput often makes the surface read younger because repair finally has the energy to keep up.

Essential fats change texture from the inside. Super Omega 3D concentrates EPA and DHA—the omega-3s that become specialized pro-resolving mediators (SPMs). These mediators tell your immune system the battle is over so healing can complete. When the inflammatory fire stops smoldering, redness fades, acne is less angry, and collagen breakdown slows. Omega-3s also slide into cell membranes to improve fluidity and signal quality—membranes are how cells "hear" hormones, including the hormones that direct collagen maintenance.

Stress leaves fingerprints on your face and scalp. High, erratic cortisol thins skin, worsens sebaceous activity in some, and erodes deep sleep—the repair window. Calm Day blends L-theanine (alpha-wave calm without sedation), magnesium (glycinate/taurate to quiet excitatory signaling and relax vessels), and supportive nutrients that help a wired nervous system downshift. Adrenal Restore layers gentle adaptogens—ashwagandha, rhodiola, eleuthero—with B-vitamins to normalize the cortisol slope. For those already flatlined by years of "go," AdrenaMax adds a sturdier foundation. People don't always buy these for skin, but they notice the difference in their skin when their sleep deepens and their days feel steadier.

Sex hormones are not just libido hormones; they are structural hormones. Rebalancing estrogen and progesterone in women reduces hot flashes and night sweats but also restores dermal thickness, hydration, and elasticity. Thoughtful testosterone restoration in women can lift mood, energy, and midface support while improving lean mass that frames the face; in men, optimized testosterone reduces visceral fat, supports endothelial function, and improves skin texture by improving sleep and growth hormone rhythm. DHEA—especially when low—can improve skin hydration and elasticity. Thyroid optimization (with cofactors like iodine, selenium, zinc, and iron in Thyroid Complete) brings back skin glow and hair luster by restoring protein synthesis and oil balance.

Peptides are targeted messengers that shine in aesthetics when paired with this foundation. GHK-Cu—the copper peptide—binds copper and delivers a "repair now" signal to skin cells; research suggests it can increase collagen and glycosaminoglycan synthesis, improve elasticity, and speed wound repair. As a topical serum, it pairs well with gentle cleansers and antioxidants; as part of comprehensive internal support, it complements collagen building and microcirculation work. Glow blends that combine GHK-Cu with BPC-157 and TB500 aim to address both surface signaling and deeper tissue calm—BPC-157 supports angiogenesis and tissue protection, while TB500 helps cells migrate efficiently to heal. KPV, a fragment of alpha-MSH, is a potent anti-inflammatory signal; for people with rosacea-like flares or sensitive, reactive skin, KPV can lower the "itchy, stingy" threshold from the inside. MOTS-C, a mitochondrial peptide, helps cells use fuel more cleanly; while often discussed for stamina and metabolism, better mitochondrial tone shows up on the skin because repair is energy-dependent. Melanotan II darkens pigment by stimulating melanocortin receptors; because it changes pigmentation and may increase the visibility of existing moles, medical supervision is essential and it is not an appearance-only toy. The point is not that peptides replace sleep, food, and hormones—they multiply the benefit of those basics when used with intention and clinical guidance.

Acne is not a teenage problem; it is an insulin, androgen, and inflammation problem that can show up at any age. High-glycemic meals spike insulin which raises IGF-1 and stimulates sebaceous glands; in women with relative androgen excess or low sex-hormone binding globulin, this effect is louder. A cross-current of gut irritation and seed-oil-heavy diets keeps the immune system on edge, so any clogged pore turns into a red, painful eruption. The fix runs through this whole chapter: steady blood sugar with protein-anchored meals and ten-minute walks after eating; rebuild the gut with IgG, Remove Complete, and GI Complete; optimize hormones (especially estrogen/progesterone balance, gentle testosterone support in women, and thyroid in both sexes); consider DIM Plus to guide estrogen metabolites down calmer pathways; use Super Omega 3D to help resolve flare; and add KPV for stubborn, inflammatory patterns. Topically, choose cleansers that leave the barrier intact, add niacinamide (for oil balance and barrier support), azelaic acid (for redness and pigment), and a vitamin C serum in the morning. Retinoids at night—retinaldehyde or retinol—improve turnover and texture. Acne calms fastest when the skin barrier is protected; over-stripping prolongs the cycle.

Pigmentation issues—melasma, sun spots, post-inflammatory marks—are hormone and inflammation stories as much as UV stories. Estrogen imbalance, pregnancy, perimenopause, and certain medications can tilt melanocyte behavior. High cortisol and chronic inflammation prime pigment cells to respond more aggressively to sunlight. Internally, steadying estrogen metabolism (DIM Plus), keeping insulin predictable, and resolving inflammation (Super Omega 3D, SPMs) change the baseline. Topically, daily mineral sunscreen (zinc and/or titanium dioxide), vitamin C, azelaic acid, niacinamide, and gentle retinoids are the long game; GHK-Cu serums can help texture look smoother even while pigment slowly evens out. Patience is the currency here—pigment loves to return if the underlying drivers remain.

Hair thinning asks for detective work, not panic. In women, ferritin (stored iron) often sits too low for robust growth even when hemoglobin is "normal"; aim for a healthy range in context with inflammation and iron saturation. Thyroid function is foundational; low free T3 will stall anagen and make hair brittle. Perimenopause adds a second layer: as estrogen drops, hair may miniaturize and shed more readily. Gentle testosterone support in women can help when energy, libido, and muscle also dip, but if acne or excess facial hair appears, re-evaluate dose and relative estrogen balance. In men, visceral fat raises aromatase, shrinking the free testosterone pool and tilting toward DHT-dominant signaling at the follicle. The inside work—protein intake, iron repletion when low, thyroid optimization, insulin control, omega-3s, and microcirculation with CircuCORE—creates the conditions follicles need. On the scalp, simple topicals like caffeine, rosemary, niacinamide, and peptides (including topical GHK-Cu) can support the local environment. Postpartum shedding (telogen effluvium) is common and self-limited; supportive nutrition, sleep recovery, and stress rhythm shorten the trough.

Topical routines should serve biology, not fight it. Morning can be as minimal as cleanse-(or rinse-only if not needed), vitamin C (L-ascorbic acid or a gentle derivative), niacinamide, and mineral sunscreen. Evening is cleanse, hydrating layers (hyaluronic acid, glycerin, panthenol), barrier support (ceramides, cholesterol, fatty acids), then your active (retinoid, copper peptides—often on alternate nights to avoid ingredient clashes). GHK-Cu plays well in hydrating, slightly acidic routines but is best not layered directly with strong acids or peroxides. Acne-prone skin tolerates azelaic acid beautifully; rosacea-prone skin prefers fewer steps, more barrier. The best routine is the one you will do—consistently. Products are support crew. Your food, sleep, stress, and hormones are the stars.

"Did you know?" Your skin's "glow" after a workout is nitric oxide, heat-shock proteins, and increased dermal blood flow talking to one another. That temporary flush isn't just cosmetic; it's a signal to fibroblasts to build better collagen. Pair that with vitamin C intake and adequate protein within a reasonable window and you are literally feeding the signal.

Nutraceuticals round out the plan by delivering what food can't always supply at therapeutic levels. Super B—the methylated B-complex—drives neurotransmitter production (you feel it as brighter mood and calmer focus), powers methylation for hormone and toxin metabolism, and supports energy enzymes that fuel repair. ADK10 pairs vitamins A, D3, and K2 to support epidermal renewal, immune rhythm, and calcium placement away from vessels and into bone. Super Omega 3D changes membrane fluidity and pushes inflammation toward resolution; when skin is red and tight, that biochemical pivot matters. Mag Complete combines high-absorption magnesium forms to relax vessels, deepen sleep, and support collagen-sparing recovery. Essential Minerals ensures zinc (critical for repair and acne control) shows up alongside copper (critical for collagen cross-linking) so the two stay in balance; selenium supports thyroid hormone activation. Thyroid Complete provides iodine, selenium, zinc, and other cofactors for graceful thyroid conversion. EnerCoQ10 and EnerDMG lift mitochondrial throughput so repair can keep pace with life. IgG, Remove Complete, ParaKill, CandiKill, and GI Complete repair the gut terrain so your face stops broadcasting immune static. CircuCORE improves microcirculation so the nutrients you take arrive where you want them—dermis and follicles. Calm Day, Adrenal Restore, and AdrenaMax recalibrate the cortisol rhythm that either steals from beauty sleep or gives it back.

Safety and sanity matter. Vitamin A should be used thoughtfully in women who are or may become pregnant. Biotin at very high doses can interfere with certain lab assays (thyroid, troponin); moderate use is plenty when the rest of the system is in place. Copper and zinc must be balanced. Peptides should be sourced through reputable medical channels that verify purity and sterility; "research grade" from random sellers is a gamble you don't need to take. Mineral sunscreens are your friend; daily use is the most reliable topical anti-aging step available and it doesn't fight your physiology—it protects it. The goal is not perfection; it is consistency with honest inputs.

If your mirror has been giving you news you don't like, take it as a prompt, not a verdict. The face and scalp you want are a downstream effect of the biology you build. Give your gut thirty days of focused care. Anchor meals with protein and color. Swap seed-oil-heavy packaged foods for olive oil, avocado, nuts, and clean proteins. Restore sleep to seven and a half to nine hours with a consistent wake time and dimmed lights at night. Optimize hormones so collagen receives the "keep building" signal again. Add nutraceuticals to cover the gaps and peptides to multiply the effect. Choose a simple topical routine and do it daily. In six weeks, you won't just see a difference—you'll feel the system that created it.

That is aesthetic longevity: beauty as a side effect of health. When your biology runs, your surface tells the truth.

Chapter 20

The Longevity Blueprint: Turn Your Plan Into a Life You Can Live

The people who age well don't rely on luck. They build a system that keeps paying them back—on good days, on travel days, and on the days when life doesn't go to plan. They aren't chasing hacks; they're running a rhythm. They know which dials to touch first, how long to keep them there, and how to notice early when something needs to change. This chapter is about turning everything you've learned into a living blueprint—one that feels human, not heroic; precise, not perfectionistic; sustainable, not fragile. It's the operating system under your choices so you don't need to wake up every morning and reinvent your health from scratch.

The first step is deciding what you are optimizing for, and "weight" is not the answer. Weight can move while health doesn't, and health can improve while weight takes its time. The targets that make a life better are the ones you feel all day long: mornings that start clear without a fight, work that requires focus without a crash, movement that leaves you charged instead of wiped out, relationships that get your patience and your presence, and evenings where sleep is a friend you can count on. Those experiences come from the interplay of four domains—signals (hormones), structure (muscle and bone), power (mitochondria and metabolic flexibility), and calm (nervous-system balance and inflammation). When you organize your plan around those four, the rest of the metrics follow.

Start with signals. Biology listens when messages are clear and delivered at the right volume. That's the quiet power of properly supervised bioidentical hormone therapy: it restores signal quality. The goal isn't to force numbers into a box; it's to return your body to the range where it recognizes itself. When messages are crisp, you notice it everywhere you live—less friction at the joints, a steadier mood, faster recovery, and that welcome sense that effort works again. Signals are also sensitive to context. If your evenings run hot with stress and blue light, progesterone's calm will feel distant. If your meals spike and crash all day, thyroid's tempo will never feel steady. Your blueprint respects both the prescription and the terrain.

Then build structure. Muscle and bone are your body's physical savings accounts. They protect you when life delivers a surprise—illness, surgery, a hard season—and they let you say "yes" to what you care about without negotiating with pain. You don't need to train like an athlete to protect them; you need to train like someone who intends to keep living independently for a very long time. Two or three sessions a week of progressive resistance—hinge, squat pattern, push, pull, carry—will keep returning dividends when your signals are optimized and your recovery is protected. Bone listens to load and impact. Muscle listens to tension and protein. Both listen to sleep.

Power is the part most people feel but struggle to name. It's the difference between a day that grinds and a day that flows. Power is your mitochondria deciding whether today's inputs get turned into energy or noise. You improve it by how you eat, how you move, and how you sleep—and you can accelerate it with targeted support when it fits your picture. The plan that works doesn't swing between restriction and indulgence; it lives mostly in the middle with meals that anchor you (protein forward, colorful plants, healthy fats) and movement that keeps your engine flexible (walking often, some intervals scaled to your season, strength that respects your joints). When power improves, the "I deserve it" late-night snacks lose their pull not because you got stricter, but because your body is no longer asking you to medicate fatigue with sugar.

Calm is not a personality trait here; it's a physiologic state. A nervous system that can accelerate and decelerate on demand is the hidden architecture of healthy aging. If your evenings feel like a bad radio station—static, volume up, hard to tune—the rest of your blueprint will skid. Your plan earns calm with early daylight, stress boundaries you can keep, breath that you actually enjoy doing, protein and magnesium at dinner, a cooler, darker room, and lights down before your brain decides to stay up without you. That may sound soft, but it's the hard wiring that lets hormones work, training stick, and appetite behave.

You do not have to build this all at once. The most successful blueprints start with an on-ramp—a deliberate four-week period where you make a few choices non-negotiable and let everything else be "nice to have." In week one, hold wake time steady, go outside early, and anchor a protein-first breakfast within two hours of waking. In week two, add two strength sessions you can actually attend and ten-minute walks after your two biggest meals. In week three, commit to a lights-down hour and move caffeine earlier. In week four, layer in your first precision levers—whether that's starting BHRT based on your labs, introducing a targeted nutraceutical foundation, or planning a short peptide cycle to support sleep or tissue repair. Four weeks is short enough to see change and long enough for a nervous system to trust you're serious.

Blueprints earn their name by telling you what to do when life pushes back. You can plan for that too. Create a "floor plan" for tough weeks—two choices for breakfast you can make in five minutes, a ten-minute at-home strength circuit that hits the big patterns, a wind-down you can do in a hotel room, and a small kit you keep ready with your essentials so travel doesn't become an excuse for chaos. Keep one bottle of a bioavailable magnesium for nights, an omega-3 you tolerate with your first meal, and a methylated B complex for busy weeks. If your hormones are part of your plan, set calendar reminders for refills and lab checks so gaps don't happen by accident. If peptides are in the mix, schedule cycles around seasons of need—sleep-supportive blends during crunch time, tissue-repair support when training adds load—then leave space off.

Data matters. But the right data. You do not need to drown in numbers to steer well. Choose a handful of measures that reflect your four domains and revisit them regularly. For signals, that means labs at sensible intervals—comprehensive sex hormone panels, a complete thyroid picture, DHEA-S, fasting insulin with glucose and A1C, vitamin D, ferritin, CRP. For structure, keep an honest strength log with the movements that matter and, when possible, periodic body-composition snapshots that distinguish muscle from everything else. For power, track a few real-life outputs: how often you wake before your alarm, whether you need caffeine to feel human, whether a brisk walk still lifts you or drags you. For calm, use the simplest check-ins: sleep continuity, time to fall asleep, your "feel" thirty minutes after a stressor (spinning or steady). Once a week, on the same day, ask the same questions. When the trend slips, adjust one dial, not ten.

One of the most helpful parts of a working blueprint is understanding what to expect and when. Early wins often show up in sleep continuity and morning clarity before the mirror budges. That's not a disappointment; that's the foundation you need for composition to follow. The next layer is training response—you'll notice soreness resolves faster and sessions feel more productive. Appetite normalizes. Mood gets smoother. Then body shape begins to change with the same work. If you start BHRT, most people feel the edges soften within weeks, while structural benefits like bone preservation accrue quietly over months and years. If you cycle peptides for sleep or repair, the best sign they're doing their job is not fireworks; it's the way your day stops feeling like a fight. Precision nutraceuticals are like bolts in a bridge: you don't notice them until they're missing. Keep them boring and consistent, and they will keep everything else from rattling loose.

Plateaus are not failure; they're feedback. When progress stalls, resist the urge to add complexity. Look for friction. Is sleep drifting later? Did protein slip? Did walking shrink because the weather changed? Did your training stop progressing because you've been lifting the same loads for months? Did you push intervals hard for three weeks and never deload? Are you drinking more at night because you're rewarding yourself for hard days? Is your dose of hormone now ahead of your plan because your body changed and you didn't update it? The reason a blueprint works is because it makes these questions easy to ask and answer. Adjust one thing. Give it time. Re-test. Move again.

There's a human part to this that rarely gets discussed: identity. People who age well don't just collect tools; they adopt a stance. They see themselves as builders, not passengers. That shift matters when life throws you something heavy. A builder doesn't negotiate with their sleep because tomorrow requires them. A builder doesn't punish themselves with exercise; they train for the life they want. A builder doesn't moralize food; they ask what job this meal needs to do and choose accordingly. And a builder doesn't make every change alone. They recruit their home to help—a darker bedroom, a calmer evening routine, a kitchen that makes the right choice easier than the wrong one, a partner who walks after dinner. Biology happens in community. Your plan will be lighter if the people closest to you know what you're trying to do and how to help.

Sourcing and safety earn a permanent place in the blueprint. Work with professionals who listen to how you live, not just to your lab report. If you use hormones, use bioidentical forms, personalize the dose, and confirm with lived results and periodic labs that you're in the physiologic window where benefits live and side effects don't. If you use peptides, use reputable medical channels with identity and purity verified; cycle them for purposes and then stop. If you use nutraceuticals, insist on transparency and third-party testing; choose forms your body can use and combinations that make sense for your picture. And keep your plan under review. The dose that helped you get out of a hole may not be the dose you need to stay well once you're strong again. The supplements that filled gaps six months ago may be replaceable with food and rhythm today. Good plans shrink when they can.

It helps to imagine your next year in chapters, not just weeks. The first ninety days are about building the base—sleep you can trust, meals that make you steady, training that rehabs your confidence, signals returned to your personal range. Months four through six are about consolidating and nudging—progressive strength, some faster walking or intervals scaled to your joints, a mitochondria-friendly rhythm that replaces long sitting with micro-movement, thoughtful adjustments to your hormone plan, and the smallest stack of targeted supplements that keep things quiet. The second half of the year is about your ambitions—adventures you want your body to say yes to, numbers you want to improve because they unlock choices later (bone density, grip strength, travel stamina), and skills that make your plan lighter: cooking a few default meals, carrying your sleep routine on the road, learning to de-escalate stress in the middle of your day instead of after it.

As you move through that year, certain transitions deserve special choreography. If you're approaching perimenopause or menopause, treat sleep as your anchor and steadiness as your friend. Use nighttime progesterone thoughtfully; choose routes of estradiol that deliver benefits without unnecessary detours; consider physiologic female doses of testosterone when drive and training traction fade. If you're in andropause, avoid the mistake of expecting training alone to overcome years of low signals; restore testosterone to a range your body recognizes and balance it with the rest of the orchestra. If you're recovering from a long fatigue season—illness, overwork, grief—don't hijack your nervous system with intensity. Rebuild with rhythm: eat, lift modestly, walk, sleep, support repair, and let desire for more arrive on its own. If your gut has been a saboteur, make calm there your first project; you can't absorb a plan you can't digest.

The blueprint also respects seasons of celebration. Holidays, big family events, travel to places you've dreamed about—these are not threats to your plan; they are why you have one. Decide in advance which non-negotiables you're taking with you (wake time, daylight, walking, protein with breakfast, your sleep kit), which negotiables you'll flex (dessert at the celebration, smaller portions of everything else), and which stories you won't tell yourself (that you "blew it," that you "have to make up for it," that the plan is "off"). Leave the trip with the same number of dials you arrived with and your body will not punish you for living.

There will be moments when you wonder whether it's worth the attention. Remember what you're buying with this consistency: a brain that keeps up with your life, joints that move without protest, a metabolism that forgives, intimacy that returns as a kindness rather than a chore, lab reports that confirm what your days already told you, and a future self that thanks you out loud. We use the word "longevity" as if it belongs to someday. In practice, longevity is your Tuesday afternoon—how you feel in it, what you can ask of it, and how much of it you have left after you've done what matters.

If you need a place to begin tomorrow, make it small and stubborn. Wake at the same time. Step outside early. Eat a protein-forward breakfast. Walk after two meals. Lift twice this week. Dim a house, not a screen. Take the magnesium you meant to take. Put your labs on a calendar and honor them like appointments with your future. If you're already doing those, choose the next precise lever based on your picture: adjust a dose, cycle a peptide for sleep or repair, address the gut you've been ignoring, or make your training progress again by adding five pounds to the bar or five minutes to the walk. Keep your plan personal, data-informed, seasonally adjusted, and boring enough to repeat. That is what turns knowledge into capacity, and capacity into a life.

Most of all, keep your compass pointed away from managed decline and toward created health. The medication-first model has a place in emergencies, but it is a poor architect for the next decade of your life. A blueprint that respects signals, structure, power, and calm—and earns them with daily choices you can keep—will make you feel younger than the math says you are. That feeling is not a trick. It's biology remembering itself. And once you've felt it, you will not want to go back.

Chapter 21

The Wellness Wake-Up: How Food, Pharma, and Policy Shaped Your Hormones—and How to Take Them Back

You were never meant to spend midlife juggling a pillbox and a calendar of specialist visits. Yet many of us are living in bodies that feel older than our birth year suggests: energy that fades by afternoon, sleep that never quite restores, brain fog, stubborn weight, erratic cycles, low libido, joint aches, and moods on a hair-trigger. We're told this is "normal aging," but the pattern starts far earlier—often in childhood—and follows us through the decades. The honest explanation is simpler and harder: we've grown up immersed in a web of hormone-active chemicals and ultra-processed inputs that our biology was never designed to navigate. When your environment whispers the wrong instructions to your cells—every single day for years—your endocrine system adapts in ways that look an awful lot like modern "aging." The fix is not a single pill; it's a strategic course correction that removes the static, restores the signal, and rebuilds capacity from the cell up. That's what this chapter helps you do.

The science community has a name for the chemical interference we're talking about: endocrine-disrupting chemicals, or EDCs—substances that can mimic, block, or scramble hormone signaling at very low doses. Major medical and scientific groups have spent over a decade mapping out the implications for reproduction, metabolism, thyroid function, neurodevelopment, and more. Their bottom line is consistent: exposures are widespread, effects are plausible to proven depending on the chemical, and reducing exposure—especially in pregnancy and childhood—makes sense while policy catches up.

Most of us encounter EDCs not as lab names, but as familiar products and habits. The plastic cup that softens in the dishwasher. The lipstick with staying power. The "fresh linen" room spray. The wrinkle-resistant sheet set. The takeout box that doesn't leak grease. The nonstick pan that never sticks. The citrus soda, neon sports drink, or fruit-colored snack. The problem isn't any one thing—it's the total load, repeated daily, across the lifespan. If you want a clear path off this treadmill, it helps to see how exposure typically unfolds, stage by stage.

In early childhood, diet and packaging matter more than most parents realize. Colorful, kid-friendly foods often come with dyes, preservatives, and plastic contact that add chemical "noise" to a small body learning to regulate itself. Pediatric leaders have flagged concerns with certain food additives and packaging chemicals—think bisphenols like BPA and phthalates—because children are uniquely vulnerable while organs and hormone systems are wiring up. Their policy advice boils down to minimizing ultra-processed products, heating food in glass or stainless rather than plastic, and choosing fresher, simpler ingredients whenever possible.

By grade school and the teen years, the exposure map shifts toward personal-care products, snacks, and school materials. Fragrance is a big one: U.S. labels can legally list dozens of fragrance compounds simply as "fragrance" or "parfum," which makes it hard for families to identify specific chemicals to avoid. Phthalates are often used to help scents linger, and parabens serve as preservatives; both have hormone activity in lab and human studies, and both commonly show up in teens who use multiple products daily. The encouraging news is that even a brief switch to low-chemical cosmetics has been shown to lower biomarker levels for phthalates, parabens, triclosan, and certain UV filters within days—proof that your choices matter and that the body wants to offload this stuff when you stop adding more.

Late teens and young adulthood add campus life, fast food, and convenience to the mix. That means more grease-resistant wrappers and boxes—historically a source of PFAS, the "forever chemicals" used for stain and water resistance. The U.S. has recently completed a voluntary phase-out of PFAS in food-contact grease-proofing, a positive step that shows policy can move when pressure builds. But PFAS are still common in stain-resistant textiles and performance clothing, so the day-to-day strategy is to eat fresh, skip grease-proof wrappers when you can, and treat "stain-resistant" fabric claims with skepticism if hormone and immune health are priorities.

By the time many people hit the 20s and 30s, a new pattern emerges: "wired-and-tired" days, light sleep, cravings, and stress-eating that pushes them toward ultra-processed calories. Add in microplastics and nanoplastics from bottled beverages—an exposure pathway that's only just becoming visible with better detection methods—and you've got a steady, subtle drip of environmental stressors. One recent analysis found bottled water can contain on the order of a hundred thousand or more tiny plastic particles per liter; the health implications are still being clarified, but prudence favors using home filtration and reusable stainless or glass where feasible.

In the 30s and 40s, fertility and metabolic resilience sit on a knife's edge. Real-world studies and reviews have connected higher exposures to certain plastics and plasticizers with markers of insulin resistance and with reproductive diagnoses like PCOS. Associations are not destiny, but they are signals to reduce load where you can—especially if cycles are irregular, symptoms line up with estrogen dominance, or insulin markers are creeping. If you've been told "your labs are normal" but your symptoms scream otherwise, it may not be your willpower; it may be the chemistry around you turning up metabolic friction just enough to matter.

Perimenopause and andropause reveal the pattern in high definition. As estrogen, progesterone, and testosterone naturally drift, the body becomes more sensitive to the quality of its inputs. Flame retardants embedded in old foam cushions or electronics casings can migrate into house dust and have been tied to thyroid disruption. Stain-guarded carpets or wrinkle-resistant clothing may trade convenience for chronic exposure to PFAS or formaldehyde-based resins. Fragranced detergents and fabric softeners can ride your linens and clothes all day long, adding inhalation and skin exposure to the lineup. No one is saying you need to live in a lab; the practical move is to swap in low-emission foam when you replace furniture, vacuum with a HEPA filter, choose "fragrance-free" over "unscented," and wash new textiles before first use. These small decisions trim your total load and make your hormone-restoration efforts work better, faster.

Menopause and later life bring another reality: the brain, bones, vessels, and muscles are all exquisitely hormone-sensitive. If you spent decades inhaling, ingesting, and absorbing low-dose disruptors, you may enter these years with a less flexible endocrine network. That's one reason BHRT can feel like taking off a weighted vest—it restores the body's master messages so tissues can respond again. But the best results appear when BHRT is paired with exposure reduction and cell-supportive nutrition; otherwise, you're asking your system to thrive while still pushing uphill against the same chemical headwinds.

If you're wondering why this situation feels worse here than in some other places, part of the answer is regulatory differences. The European Union lowered its tolerable daily intake for BPA dramatically in 2023 and has moved to ban BPA broadly from food-contact materials; it banned BPA in baby bottles years ago and restricted its use in thermal receipt paper. The EU also tightened rules on several common phthalates in consumer products, and it has removed certain whitening additives from foods entirely. U.S. policy has improved in spots—for example, eliminating BPA in baby bottles and completing the phase-out of PFAS in greasable food packaging—but it's still typical for American consumers to shoulder more label reading and self-defense than their European counterparts. The takeaway isn't to fear your pantry; it's to buy more foods without barcodes, heat in glass or stainless, and treat packaging and fragrance claims with healthy skepticism.

Here's why all of this leads straight back to hormone optimization. Hormones are the operating system for your body. When the OS is clean and well-tuned, your cells interpret the world accurately. When the OS is constantly interrupted by decoy signals, the hardware works harder and wears faster. Removing decoys—choosing food that is food, swapping scented for fragrance-free, upgrading cookware, ditching "wrinkle-free" in favor of breathable natural fibers—turns down the static so BHRT can do its job: restore the instruction set that tells your tissues to repair, rebuild, and regulate.

As your environment gets cleaner, medical-grade nutraceuticals become the leverage that fills gaps fast. Not all supplements are created equal. Professional-grade B-complex (methylated) supports the enzyme systems that drive mitochondrial energy and hormone metabolism. Magnesium anchors ATP stability and calms over-firing nerves. Omega-3s help keep cell and mitochondrial membranes flexible. CoQ10 moves electrons along the mitochondrial chain and stabilizes membranes in high-energy tissues. Targeted botanicals and immunoglobulins can support gut barrier integrity—the front door for many exposures—so fewer irritants reach circulation. Quality here means identity, purity, and potency testing that matches what clinicians rely on in practice; the corner-store multi isn't built for the job.

There's also a place for peptides in cleaning up downstream effects of exposure. MOTS-C nudges cells toward better metabolic flexibility through AMPK-linked pathways. BPC-157 and KPV help settle inflammation and support gut repair, particularly useful if your lifetime of exposure has left you with digestive symptoms and nutrient malabsorption. None of these erase the need to take out the trash at the source, but they do accelerate the rebuild once you've done so.

If you want a practical, low-drama way to start, think in two-week sprints. In your kitchen, replace most packaged snacks with nuts, seeds, fruit, plain yogurt, olives, and simple proteins you cook once and reheat. Shift coffee out of plastic pods and into stainless or glass; brew water through a reputable filter. Eat hot foods from glass or ceramic, not warm plastic. On your skin and hair, favor short ingredient lists and products that are explicitly fragrance-free; if you wear perfume, use it on clothing you'll launder rather than directly on skin. In your home, open windows when cleaning, vacuum with a HEPA filter, and turn down the "scent marketing" you've been sold. Wash new sheets and shirts before sleeping in them; if a tag says "wrinkle-free," it likely earned that label by chemical means. None of this requires perfection. It requires momentum.

Did you know? A short, real-world teen intervention that swapped everyday cosmetics for low-chemical alternatives cut urinary levels of several hormone-active chemicals—phthalates, parabens, triclosan, and a UV filter—within just three days. If that's possible in 72 hours for teens using multiple products, imagine the cumulative benefit of cleaner inputs at every age.

There's another piece to the wake-up call: incentives. Ultra-processed foods are engineered for bliss points and shelf life, not satiety or hormone harmony. Fragranced everything creates brand signatures that ride along with you all day. Stain-resistant and wrinkle-free save time and sell units. Fee-for-service medicine rewards brief visits and prescriptions more reliably than counseling on sleep, food, and label literacy. This is not a villain story; it's an incentive story. Once you see it, you stop being surprised that your default environment fights your biology—and you stop waiting for a memo that says it's time to change.

If you're ready to rewrite your trajectory, stack your moves in this order. First, remove the loudest disruptors: ultra-processed snacks and sweet drinks; heating food in plastic; fragranced home and laundry products; nonstick pans that scratch; "stain-guarded" or "wrinkle-free" textiles against skin. Second, build a mitochondria-first lifestyle: resistance training twice weekly, brief intervals twice weekly, daily walking, regular sleep, protein-anchored meals, and daylight in your eyes morning and midday. Third, test and optimize hormones with a clinician who understands healthspan, not just lifespan; restore thyroid, sex steroids, and adrenal rhythm to optimal—not merely "normal"—ranges. Fourth, add precision support: medical-grade B-complex, magnesium, omega-3s, CoQ10, and any targeted gut or cognitive supports your history indicates. Finally, consider peptide cycles that match your goals—metabolic flexibility, recovery, gut lining, or cognitive edge.

This is how you flip the script that Big Food and the pharmaceutical business model quietly thrive on. They profit when you stay in the gray zone—never well enough to be off the carousel, never "sick enough" to be pushed into root-cause care. You won't win that game by outrage alone. You win by building a life where your baseline diet, daily movement, sleep rhythm, home air, skin products, and fabrics add up to fewer mixed messages for your hormones. Then BHRT, peptides, and real food deliver what they're capable of: strength, clarity, stable moods, better sleep, and a metabolism that behaves like it belongs to a younger person.

The larger system will continue to evolve. Regulators are reevaluating tolerable intakes for legacy chemicals; states are banning additives that nations abroad removed years ago; federal agencies have begun phasing some problem chemicals out of food contact entirely. Those are good signals, but policy always lags biology. Your cells live in real time. Choose the cleanest inputs available to you now, and watch what happens when the noise drops and the signal returns. That's not optimism. That's physiology.

Chapter 22

The Wellness Future: Breaking Free from Big Pharma's Model

The future of medicine will not arrive in a plastic bottle with a childproof cap. It will not be defined by waiting rooms filled with people who have grown used to being told their symptoms are "normal for your age." The future of medicine lives in kitchens where meals are built around protein and color, in bedrooms where lights dim early and sleep runs deep, in gyms where strength is treated like a vital sign, and inside clinics that measure progress by healthspan instead of refill counts. The Wellness Future is not an abstract idea; it's already being lived by people who decided to stop outsourcing their biology and start leading it.

People stay trapped in "managed decline" because the traditional model fragments problems and sells parts. A pill for blood pressure here, something for reflux there, a sedative for sleep, a stimulant for the morning crash—and still no answer to the question that matters: why is the system underperforming? Your body is not a collection of unrelated complaints; it is an orchestra. When the conductor's signals (your hormones) fade, when the strings (mitochondria) are out of tune, when the percussion (nervous system) plays erratic, when the room acoustics (gut and vasculature) distort the sound, the song of your health falls apart. The Wellness Future puts the sections back in time and tune.

The first move in the Wellness Future is to end the myth that symptoms must be "tolerated" because of a birth date. Fatigue is not a personality trait. Brain fog is not a character flaw. Midsection weight is not a moral failure. These are signals that the system wants attention—signals you can answer. You answer them by restoring rhythm to your days and nights, then repairing the terrain those days and nights shape. Sleep becomes the nightly meeting where repair gets assigned. Morning light, a consistent wake time, and an evening wind-down ritual restore your cortisol slope and your growth-hormone pulses. With that rhythm set, everything else gets easier because your biology finally has a schedule to keep.

The next move is to reset the gut, because your digestive tract is the switchboard that routes signals everywhere else. A porous gut leaks fragments of microbial cell walls into circulation; your immune system hears danger and inflames tissues that are thin and richly innervated—joints, skin, brain, vascular endothelium. You feel it as bloating by evening, achy hands after certain meals, a face that flushes too easily, or a mood that turns irritable without warning. A focused "remove and repair" phase changes the terrain fast. Remove ultra-processed foods and common irritants for four to eight weeks. Bind and neutralize what shouldn't be there with serum-derived IgG, support tight-junction integrity with glutamine and zinc-carnosine, and calm the immune cross-talk in the gut wall with KPV. If clinical history suggests overgrowths, short targeted seasons with botanicals (e.g., oregano, berberine blends) or specific formulas to address parasites or candida can be useful under guidance. As the gut quiets, insulin sensitivity improves, cortisol steadies, and the skin/brain/joints stop getting daily alarm calls.

With rhythm and terrain set, hormones become the conductors again. Bioidentical replacement is not about making a lab look "young"; it is about restoring the messages that tell tissues to build, repair, and protect. Estradiol supports synapses, vasodilation, and glucose handling in the brain; progesterone deepens sleep and steadies the nervous system via GABAergic pathways; testosterone—yes, in women as well as men—drives protein synthesis, motivation, and recovery; thyroid hormones set the tempo in every cell; DHEA is the buffer that aids immune balance and stress adaptation. Optimizing these signals does not replace lifestyle; it multiplies the return on your effort. People notice they can train, digest, think, and sleep like their investment finally "lands."

Peptides sit alongside BHRT as the precision tools that remove bottlenecks and speed repair. They are short amino-acid messengers that nudge the pathways your body already built. Some restore youthful growth-hormone pulsatility so you recover from training and sleep more deeply (CJC-1295 with Ipamorelin; Sermorelin). Others accelerate soft-tissue and gut repair (BPC-157, TB500, KPV). Mitochondrial-support peptides (MOTS-C with AICAR) remind cells how to make ATP with less friction, and neuro-cognitive blends (e.g., NAD+ with BDNF and choline donors) sharpen focus and memory. When used in time-bound cycles and paired with sleep, protein, and training, they behave like accelerators—not magic, just smart physiology.

Food is not just fuel in this future; it is the daily script your biology reads. The same calories, in different forms, write wildly different stories. Protein first at meals gives your immune system amino acids to rebuild and your muscles the signal to grow. Color—greens, brassicas, berries, herbs—delivers polyphenols that cool oxidative stress and support the liver and microbiome pathways that metabolize hormones safely. Healthy fats from olive oil, avocado, nuts, and cold-water fish become the membranes your cell receptors live in; better membranes hear hormone signals more clearly. This is why people feel different on the same calories but higher quality—because the information changed.

Nutraceuticals are strategic in the Wellness Future because food, while foundational, does not always supply therapeutic levels of the cofactors your plan relies on. The goal is precision, not a pile of bottles. Think "ingredients with jobs." A methylated B-complex (Super B) provides folate as 5-MTHF and B12 as methylcobalamin for methylation, P-5-P (active B6) for neurotransmitters, riboflavin and niacin for mitochondrial dehydrogenases—people feel this as brighter morning energy and calmer focus. Vitamins A, D3, and K2 (ADK10) work like traffic control for calcium and receptor integrity—supporting bone, vascular flexibility, immune rhythm, and hormone receptor function. High-potency omega-3s (Super Omega 3D) supply EPA/DHA to brighten membranes and become specialized pro-resolving mediators (SPMs)—the "off switch" for inflammation—so tissues can heal completely instead of smoldering. DIM Plus shapes estrogen metabolism toward favorable pathways in women and men. GI repair blends deliver glutamine, zinc-carnosine, and botanicals to rebuild the wall;

serum-derived IgG binds microbial antigens that don't belong. Magnesium in well-absorbed forms (glycinate, malate, taurate) calms the nervous system, supports heart rhythm, and deepens sleep. Daytime calm formulas (with L-theanine, taurine, magnesium) help you be steady without sedation; adaptogen blends range from gentle (ashwagandha, rhodiola, eleuthero) to robust, normalizing the cortisol slope when life runs hot.

Circulation is the delivery system for every good choice you make, so vascular tone becomes a pillar in this model. Nitric oxide (NO) is the molecule your endothelium uses to tell vessels to relax; under stress, inactivity, hyperglycemia, or sleep loss, NO fades and tissues do not receive what they need. A comprehensive vascular formula can supply the chemistry your endothelium uses to generate and protect NO: vitamin C to shield the signal and support collagen in vessel walls; methylated folate (Quatrefolic®) to recycle homocysteine and reduce endothelial friction; beet-root nitrates to be converted to NO; L-citrulline and L-arginine as substrates; and polyphenols such as grape-seed OPCs and hawthorn to preserve elasticity. People feel the payoff as warmer hands and feet, friendlier blood pressure, clearer thinking during the afternoon, and better exercise tolerance—because oxygen delivery improved.

Energy is the rate-limiting step for most modern lives, and mitochondria pay that bill. Coenzyme Q10 is a literal electron shuttle in the respiratory chain and a membrane stabilizer; providing it in meaningful doses supports cardiac and skeletal muscle output, especially for people on statins or anyone who notices "lag" under higher training loads. Dimethylglycine functions as an indirect methyl donor and a metabolic buffer; clinically, people notice steadier endurance, cleaner recovery, and calmer concentration without stimulation. Together, these inputs help you make ATP with fewer sparks—more energy, less oxidative wear.

Because this chapter is a manifesto and not a menu, it is worth saying clearly: you do not need everything at once. The Wellness Future is built by sequence and focus. Start by restoring rhythm. Then repair the gut. Then optimize hormones. Then add peptides to remove bottlenecks and accelerate gains. Support every phase with targeted nutraceuticals that match the task at hand. Measurement keeps you honest but not obsessive. Hormone panels, full thyroid assessment, fasting insulin and A1c, particle-based lipids when available, hs-CRP, ferritin in context, vitamin D, B12/folate, magnesium, and iron studies provide a clear map. If sleep is restless or blood pressure is stubborn, screen for sleep apnea. If family history is loaded for cardiovascular disease, add ApoB and (when warranted) lipoprotein(a). If cognitive drift worries you, track sleep efficiency, strength sessions completed, post-meal glucose, and practice repetition—you can measure your way back to clarity.

Clinics that embrace the Wellness Future measure what matters and design care around repeatable wins. They start visits with sleep and light, not just labs. They make muscle a metric. They teach simple meal anchors and pair them with ten-minute post-meal walks. They sequence care—sleep and gut first, hormones second, peptides third—and they document outcomes that are easy to feel and easy to defend: blood pressure softens, fasting insulin drops, A1c falls, triglycerides normalize, hs-CRP cools, ferritin lands in a healthy range, strength rises, VO_2 improves, sleep deepens, libido returns. They choose medical-grade nutraceuticals that match the chemistry discussed above, and they source peptides through channels that verify content and sterility. The result is a clinic measured by healthspan—not prescription volume.

Employers can join this future by shifting incentives from copays on sick-care to benefits for sleep, strength, and insulin sensitivity. Changing a workplace culture looks mundane on paper: dark-mode evenings, morning light breaks, a real lunch, walking meetings, and access to basic lab panels tied to coaching. On the balance sheet, it looks like fewer absences, sharper teams, less burnout, and lower long-term costs. Communities can participate by making healthy food more available than fast food, building safe, lit walking paths, and supporting school curricula that prioritize movement, light, and real food over screens and sugar.

Safety and quality are part of that scale. Bioidentical hormones should be individualized and monitored; the goal is function, not excess. Peptides must come through reputable medical channels that verify purity and sterility; counterfeits and contaminants are a bridge you never need to cross. Nutraceuticals should be third-party tested and formulated with the forms your body recognizes—methylfolate over folic acid, methylcobalamin over cyanocobalamin, chelated minerals over salts. Cheap supplements that don't move biology are the most expensive kind—because they cost you time.

Did you know that your cells "hear" hormones through receptors embedded in membranes made from the fats you eat? Diets rich in extra-virgin olive oil, avocado, nuts, and cold-water fish build more fluid, responsive membranes than diets dominated by industrial seed oils. That single detail is one reason omega-3 intake and fat quality show up across this book—from cardiovascular flexibility to brain clarity to sex-hormone sensitivity. Your receptors are listening; give them a surface that delivers the message.

If you are a reader holding this book and wondering where to begin, start tonight. Dim the lights an hour before bed. Put your phone in another room. Take magnesium and write down three things you will do tomorrow that match this plan. Eat a protein-anchored breakfast. Walk after lunch. Lift something with good form. Drink water. Go to bed a little earlier. Order labs and review them with someone who understands optimization, not just symptom control. Choose one peptide cycle that addresses your biggest bottleneck. Track simple wins: sleep through, afternoon energy, smoother workouts. Celebrate them.

If you are a clinician, the invitation is to build your practice around momentum. Teach rhythm first. Make a short gut-repair season standard. Use BHRT to restore signal, not chase numbers. Layer peptides in time-bound cycles to solve real problems and then pause. Document outcomes with the labs that matter and the metrics people feel. Build a simple nutraceutical formulary grounded in ingredient chemistry: methyl donors and mitochondrial cofactors in the morning; omega-3s and vitamin D/K2 for membranes and resolution; magnesium at night. Educate every patient that sleep and strength are non-negotiables. Then deliver follow-up systems that keep the wins compounding.

If you are an employer or community leader, start with light, sleep, movement, and food. Create policies that make evening emails optional, morning light normal, walking breaks encouraged, and real food accessible. Support strength training on-site or nearby. Offer simple lab panels and coaching. Celebrate healthspan metrics—sleep efficiency, steps, lifts completed, insulin sensitivity—like you celebrate quarterly wins. The Wellness Future scales because biology is universal; the details can be local.

And if you are anyone who wants to implement the supplement side of this work with trusted, medical-grade products, the options discussed throughout this book are available for purchase here: https://www.revitalizenutrition.net/shop-now. Use what matches your plan and your labs. Quality and consistency are what turn theory into outcomes.

The Wellness Future is not about chasing youth. It is about building capacity so your years are full of strength, clarity, and ease. It is about choosing inputs that make your biology generous—hormones that say "repair," peptides that remove friction, food that calms, supplements that do real jobs, sleep that restores, stress that cycles, training that tells your body you are going to need it tomorrow. The payoff is not just longer life; it is more life in your years: mornings with focus, afternoons with stamina, evenings with presence, and relationships with enough energy left over to enjoy them.

Put the book down and start with one move tonight. Momentum loves action. A week from now you will feel it. A month from now you will believe it. A year from now you will be living a different story—the one where you stopped outsourcing your health and started leading it.

Appendix A:

Nutraceutical Reference & Protocol Tables

This appendix summarizes evidence-informed nutraceuticals referenced throughout the book and organizes them into practical, clinic-neutral tables you can review with a qualified healthcare professional. Each table highlights the product purpose, key actives, how they work, and typical use notes. Doses and combinations should always be individualized based on your history, medications, labs, and goals. The listings are examples to help you understand options; they are not endorsements or prescriptions.

Important: The supplement charts, sample stacks, and dosing ranges in this book are **for reference only.** They are illustrations—not prescriptions. Do not start, stop, or change any medication, supplement, peptide, or therapy based on this book without working with a qualified healthcare professional who knows your history, medications, and labs. See the full medical disclaimer in the front matter.

A1. Foundational Health & Hormone Readiness

These build the base upon which BHRT, peptides, movement, sleep, and targeted protocols work better.

Product	Primary Focus	Key Ingredients (highlights)	How It Works (Mechanisms)	Typical Use / Notes
Women's Complete	Foundational multi for women	Activated B-complex (methylfolate/Quatrefolic®, methylcobalamin), chelated minerals (Albion®), choline (VitaCholine®), probiotics, superfoods	Covers micronutrient gaps; supports methylation, energy, hormone metabolism, cognitive & prenatal support; probiotic blend for gut/immune balance	Daily base multi; pairs with DIM Plus for estrogen metabolism; per-label dosing.
Women's Vitality	Women's performance & energy	Activated vitamins/minerals plus targeted botanicals	Supports energy, mood, thyroid/adrenal balance; complements BHRT	Daily foundational formula; per-label dosing.
Men's Complete	Foundational multi for men	Activated B-complex, chelated minerals (Albion®), antioxidants & superfoods	Fills common micronutrient gaps; supports energy, metabolism, cardiovascular health	Daily base multi; pairs with omega-3 and magnesium; per-label dosing.
Men's Vitality	Men's performance & energy	Activated vitamins/minerals plus targeted botanicals	Supports energy, hormone metabolism, stress resilience and performance	Daily foundational formula; per-label dosing.
Super B (Methyl B Complex)	Methylation & energy	5-MTHF, methylcobalamin, P5P (B6), riboflavin-5'-phosphate, biotin, pantothenic acid	Methylation support; neurotransmitter synthesis; homocysteine balance; cellular energy (ATP)	Daily with meals; helpful for fatigue, mood, detox support.
Essential Minerals	Broad mineral repletion	TRAACS® chelated minerals (Mg, Zn, Se, Cr, Mn, Mo, Cu, etc.)	Highly bioavailable minerals for enzymes, thyroid conversion, insulin sensitivity, antioxidant defenses	Daily with meals; complements multis and omega-3s.
ADK10 / ADK5	Bone, cardiovascular & hormone metabolism	Vitamin A, Vitamin D3 (10,000 IU or 5,000 IU), Vitamin K2 (MK-7)	D3/K2 synergy directs calcium to bone (away from arteries); supports immune & hormone receptor function	Select 10k or 5k IU based on labs/sunlight; caution with anticoagulants unless supervised.
Super Omega 3D	Inflammation & cardiometabolic	EPA/DHA omega-3s + Vitamin D3	Resolves inflammation, improves triglycerides, joint & brain function; D3 aids immune/hormone signaling	Take with meals; useful for pain, mood, and metabolic health.
Mag Complete 300	Magnesium repletion & relaxation	Magnesium bisglycinate, taurate, and malate (Albion®)	Cofactor in 300+ enzymes; supports muscle/nerve relaxation, sleep quality, insulin sensitivity	Evening dosing often preferred; ~300 mg/day (split doses) per label.

A2. Hormone Metabolism & Endocrine Support

Product	Primary Focus	Key Ingredients (highlights)	How It Works (Mechanisms)	Typical Use / Notes
DIM Plus	Estrogen metabolism balance	DIM, Calcium D-glucarate, Broccoli/Sulforaphane	Promotes favorable 2-hydroxy estrogen pathways; supports detox of xenoestrogens	Useful in estrogen dominance, PMS/perimenopause; for men on T to balance estradiol.
DHEA	Adrenal & androgen precursor	Micronized DHEA	Supports mood, libido, immune balance; counter-regulatory to stress	Use only with lab monitoring; start low; morning dosing.
Thyroid Complete	Thyroid conversion & signaling	Iodine, selenium, zinc, tyrosine, ashwagandha, B-vitamins	Cofactors for T4→T3 conversion and receptor sensitivity; supports metabolism & hair/skin	Pair with protein-forward diet and magnesium; monitor thyroid labs.

A3. Stress, Adrenal Rhythm & Sleep

Product	Primary Focus	Key Ingredients (highlights)	How It Works (Mechanisms)	Typical Use / Notes
Calm Day	Daytime calm focus	GABA, Glycine, Taurine, L-Theanine (Suntheanine®), P5P, B5	Increases alpha-wave relaxation; supports GABA tone and stress resilience—without sedation	1–2× daily per label; helpful for overwhelm and focus.
AdrenaMax	Adrenal adaptogen support	Ashwagandha, Rhodiola, Eleuthero, Schisandra, Vitamin C, B5, (±licorice)	Balances HPA axis; supports cortisol rhythm, stamina and recovery	AM/Noon dosing; avoid late PM; monitor BP if licorice present.
Adrenal Restore	Evening cortisol smoothing	Phosphatidylserine, ashwagandha, magnesium, L-theanine	Normalizes elevated evening cortisol to improve sleep onset and recovery	Take in evening; pairs well with Sleep Time.
Sleep Time	Sleep onset & depth	GABA, Glycine, Taurine, L-Theanine, 5-HTP, P5P, Melatonin	Supports serotonin/melatonin pathways and inhibitory neurotransmission for sleep architecture	Take 30–60 min before bed; caution with SSRIs/SNRIs (5-HTP).

A4. GI Barrier, Microbiome & Detox

Product	Primary Focus	Key Ingredients (highlights)	How It Works (Mechanisms)	Typical Use / Notes
GI Complete	Gut lining repair & digestion	L-Glutamine, aloe, DGL licorice, marshmallow, slippery elm, zinc carnosine	Soothes/rebuilds intestinal mucosa; improves absorption; reduces gut-derived inflammation	Use during gut reset; pair with IgG; take away from very hot beverages.
IgG (SBI)	Gut immune & toxin binding	Serum-derived bovine immunoglobulins	Binds LPS/endotoxins and microbial antigens; supports barrier and immune balance	Mix in cool liquids 1–2×/day; compatible with probiotics.
Remove Complete	Detox & drainage foundation	NAC, milk thistle (silymarin), alpha-lipoic acid, selenium, molybdenum, bitters	Supports liver Phase I/II, bile flow and cellular antioxidant capacity	Use during resets or exposures; hydrate well.
Para-Kill	Targeted anti-parasite herbs	Black walnut, wormwood, clove, berberine (typical)	Disrupts parasite life cycles and biofilms; antimicrobial spectrum	Structured cycles with binder support; avoid in pregnancy.
CandiKill	Yeast/candida balance	Caprylic acid, oregano, berberine, undecylenic acid	Reduces yeast overgrowth; supports microbiome rebalance	Rotate with probiotics; short courses per practitioner plan.

A5. Inflammation Resolution & Cardiovascular Support

Product	Primary Focus	Key Ingredients (highlights)	How It Works (Mechanisms)	Typical Use / Notes
SPM	Inflammation resolution mediators	Specialized pro-resolving mediators (resolvin/protectin precursors)	Promotes resolution (not suppression) of inflammation; supports post-injury recovery	Use with omega-3 base; peri-injury or chronic protocols.
X-Flame	Multi-pathway inflammation support	Kre-Celazine®, DMG HCl, turmeric (95% curcuminoids), boswellia, quercetin/rutin, ginger, cayenne	Modulates COX/LOX pathways, cytokines and joint mobility	Per-label dosing with food; pairs with Super Omega 3D.
EZ-Iron	Gentle iron repletion	TRAACS® iron bis-glycinate (Ferrochel®)	Highly bioavailable iron with less GI irritation; supports ferritin/hemoglobin	Use only if deficient; monitor ferritin and transferrin saturation.

A6. Mitochondrial & Cellular Energy

Product	Primary Focus	Key Ingredients (highlights)	How It Works (Mechanisms)	Typical Use / Notes
EnerCoQ10	Electron transport & antioxidant	Coenzyme Q10 (300 mg), Vitamin E, DMG	Supports ETC electron shuttling and membrane stability; antioxidant protection for heart/brain/muscle	With meals; consider during statin use or fatigue.*
EnerDMG	Methylation & oxygen use	N,N-Dimethylglycine (DMG)	Supports one-carbon metabolism, immune balance and cellular oxygen utilization; reduces lactic buildup	Daily or cycled around high-demand days; pairs with training.*
CircuCORE	Microcirculation & vascular health	Comprehensive circulation blend (per spec sheet)	Supports endothelial function, healthy flow and nutrient/oxygen delivery	Use for cognitive/energy support tied to circulation; per label.*

A7. Brain, Focus & Cognitive Longevity

Product	Primary Focus	Key Ingredients (highlights)	How It Works (Mechanisms)	Typical Use / Notes
BrainBoost	Multi-pathway cognitive support	Acetyl-L-carnitine, phosphatidylserine, huperzine A, bacopa, alpha-GPC	Supports acetylcholine, neuroplasticity and mitochondrial function	Morning dosing; caution with cholinergic meds.
Lion's Mane	Nerve growth factor support	Hericium erinaceus fruiting body extract	Supports neurogenesis, focus and mood via NGF pathways	Daily use; pairs with omega-3 and magnesium threonate.

A8. Cardiometabolic & Vascular Support

Product	Key Actives	How It Works	Typical Use
CircuCORE	L-citrulline, L-taurine, hawthorn, grape seed extract, bioflavonoids (per spec)	Supports endothelial nitric oxide, healthy circulation, blood pressure in normal range, and exercise tolerance	Daily; away from stimulants; monitor BP response.
Super Omega 3D	EPA/DHA (+ D3)	Triglyceride and inflammatory support; endothelial function	With meals; long-term use.
ADK10 / ADK5	A, D3, K2	Vascular calcium handling; synergistic with omega-3s and resistance training	Daily with fat; track labs.

Appendix B
Peptide Reference & Protocol Tables

This appendix summarizes the peptides referenced in the book and organizes them by primary goal (for example, body composition, recovery, sleep, cognitive support, skin and hair). Each entry provides the class/type, a plain-language mechanism, key use considerations, and practical notes to help you have informed conversations with your licensed healthcare professional. This section is clinic-neutral and strictly educational. It is not a guide to self-source or self-administer any therapy; quality, identity, and sterility require professional oversight.

Important: The supplement and peptide charts, sample stacks, and dosing ranges in this book are **for reference only**. They are illustrations—not prescriptions. Do not start, stop, or change any medication, supplement, peptide, or therapy based on this book without working with a qualified healthcare professional who knows your history, medications, and labs.

Regulatory note: Availability and regulatory status for peptides can vary by jurisdiction and may change over time. Many peptides are not approved by the U.S. Food and Drug Administration for the indications discussed. Always follow local laws and professional guidance.

B1. Sourcing & Quality (Research-Grade vs Pharmaceutical-Grade) — Quick View

Category	What It Means	Implications
Pharmaceutical-Grade	Produced under cGMP with validated identity, purity, sterility, and stability; lot traceability; prescription via licensed provider.	Highest assurance for safety/consistency; typically required for injectables; often more costly; availability varies by jurisdiction.
Research-Grade (Provider-Sourced)	Compounded or research-labeled materials from vetted labs that provide COAs and sterility testing; dispensed via medical programs.	Feasible option when pharm-grade unavailable; quality depends on source; provider oversight is essential for screening and dosing.
Research-Grade (Unverified Online)	Unknown synthesis/handling; often lacks COAs, sterility, or proper storage.	Avoid. Risk of mislabeling, contamination, incorrect concentration; legal and safety concerns.

Bottom line: work with a medical professional who uses reputable, test-verified sources. Ask for Certificates of Analysis (identity, purity, endotoxin/bioburden) and proper storage/shipping conditions.

B2. Growth Hormone Axis & Body Composition

Peptide / Blend	Primary Focus	Core Mechanism(s)	Typical Clinical Rationale	Form / Notes
CJC-1295 + Ipamorelin	GH pulse support, body comp, recovery	GHRH analog + GHSR agonist → ↑ GH pulsatility → downstream IGF-1	Support lean mass, fat loss, sleep quality, soft-tissue recovery when GH signaling is low-normal	Evening or split dosing; monitor IGF-1; avoid in active malignancy.
Sermorelin	Physiologic GH stimulation	GHRH analog → pituitary GH release within native feedback loops	Gentle GH support; early decline or younger adults	Bedtime dosing common; cycle and monitor.
Tesamorelin	Visceral fat reduction, metabolic health	Stabilized GHRH analog → ↑ GH → preferential ↓ visceral adipose tissue	Targeted VAT reduction; cardiometabolic risk support	Monitor waist/VAT & IGF-1; inject per guidance.
IGF-1 LR3	Anabolic support, hypertrophy	IGF-1 receptor agonism → ↑ protein synthesis / satellite cells	Short blocks to accelerate strength/mass with training	Medical supervision; hypoglycemia risk; cycle use.
AOD9604	Fat metabolism (non-GH)	GH 176-191 fragment → ↑ lipolysis / ↓ lipogenesis without ↑ GH/IGF-1	Adjunct for stubborn adiposity with lifestyle program	Generally well tolerated; pair with diet & training.

B3. Tissue Repair, Inflammation & Gut

Peptide / Blend	Primary Focus	Core Mechanism(s)	Typical Clinical Rationale	Form / Notes
BPC-157	Gut & musculoskeletal repair; anti-inflammatory	Cytoprotective peptide → angiogenesis, fibroblast migration; GI mucosal healing	Tendon/ligament strains, GI barrier support, overuse injuries	Often paired with TB500; source quality critical.
TB500	Tissue regeneration & mobility	Actin-binding → cell migration, angiogenesis; reduced fibrosis/inflammation	Mobility after injury, post-surgical remodeling, athletic recovery	Cycle 4–8 weeks; reassess training load.
BPC-157 + TB500	Accelerated soft-tissue repair	Synergistic angiogenesis + cytoprotection + anti-inflammatory signaling	Chronic tendinopathy, multi-site overuse, higher training volumes	Blend simplifies stacking; reassess at 4–8 weeks.
KPV	Anti-inflammatory, gut immune modulation	α-MSH tripeptide fragment → melanocortin pathway → ↓ NF-κB / cytokines	IBD-like flares, post-infectious gut irritation, skin-gut axis	Pairs with BPC-157 for lining + immune calm.
BPC / TB4 / MGF / KPV	Comprehensive repair & inflammation control	Cytoprotection + actin remodeling + mechano-growth factor + melanocortin anti-inflammatory	Complex injuries, multi-tissue recovery, repetitive strain	Simplifies stacking; reassess progress at 4–8 weeks.

B4. Mitochondrial & Metabolic Efficiency

Peptide / Blend	Primary Focus	Core Mechanism(s)	Typical Clinical Rationale	Form / Notes
MOTS-C + AICAR	Mitochondrial efficiency, endurance, glucose handling	Mitochondrial-derived peptide + AMPK activator → ↑ FA oxidation, metabolic flexibility	Low energy, deconditioning, aerobic base rebuild, weight plateau	Cycle around training blocks; caution in hypotension/hypoglycemia.

B5. Cognitive, Mood & Neuroplasticity

Peptide / Blend	Primary Focus	Core Mechanism(s)	Typical Clinical Rationale	Form / Notes
NAD+ / BDNF / Alpha GPC	Cellular energy & neuroplasticity	NAD+ for mitochondrial redox; BDNF signaling; cholinergic tone via Alpha GPC	Brain fog, focus, learning blocks; pairs with sleep & exercise	Morning use; avoid late PM.
Brain Ultra 7	Advanced nootropic stack	NAD+, Selank, Semax, BDNF, Oxytocin, Alpha GPC, Huperzine, Dihexa	High-demand cognitive periods; mood/focus; neuroplasticity goals	Medical oversight; avoid combining with other cholinesterase inhibitors.
Selank	Anxiolytic, pro-cognitive	Tuftsin analog → GABAergic modulation, neurotrophic signaling	Stressful seasons, public-facing roles, calm focus	Daytime use; pairs with magnesium and sleep hygiene.

B6. Sexual Health & Photoprotection

Peptide / Blend	Primary Focus	Core Mechanism(s)	Typical Clinical Rationale	Form / Notes
PT-141	Libido/sexual arousal (men & women)	MC4R agonist (melanocortin) → central arousal pathways	Low desire unrelated to sex hormone deficiency; adjunct to BHRT	On-demand or cyclic; common transient flushing/nausea.
Melanotan II	Tanning photoprotection; libido adjunct	MC1R/MC4R agonism → ↑ melanogenesis; central arousal effects	Fair skin photoprotection goals; libido adjunct in select cases	Potential hyperpigmentation or nausea; sun guidance essential.

B7. Aesthetic, Skin & Hair Support

Peptide / Blend	Primary Focus	Core Mechanism(s)	Typical Clinical Rationale	Form / Notes
GHK-Cu	Collagen, skin repair, hair support	Copper peptide → ↑ collagen/elastin synthesis, ECM remodeling, follicle signaling	Skin rejuvenation, scar remodeling, early hair thinning	Topical/locational common; avoid systemic copper overload.
Glow	Aesthetic healing & anti-inflammation	Tissue repair + anti-inflammation + collagen remodeling	Post-procedure recovery; aesthetic rejuvenation with less downtime	Adjunct to skincare and procedural plans; clinician-guided.

B8. Muscle, Strength & Recovery

Peptide / Blend	Class / Type	Plain-Language Mechanism	Primary Uses & Notes
IGF-1 LR3	IGF-1 analog (extended action)	Stimulates muscle protein synthesis and satellite cell activity downstream of GH/insulin pathways.	Lean mass and strength blocks; experienced users only; requires careful medical oversight (glucose monitoring).

B9. Symptom-to-Peptide Matrix

Symptom/Goal	Peptide Options (Discuss with Provider)
Slow recovery from training / tendon niggles	BPC-157; TB500; BPC-157 + TB500; KPV
IBS-like flares / leaky gut concerns	BPC-157; KPV; BPC-157/TB4/MGF/KPV blend
Stubborn visceral fat / low energy	CJC-1295 + Ipamorelin; Tesamorelin; MOTS-C + AICAR; AOD9604
Low drive / libido (men or women)	PT-141; (consider hormone optimization alongside)
Cognitive fog / high-demand work blocks	Selank; NAD+/BDNF/Alpha GPC; Brain Ultra 7
Skin elasticity / hair thinning support	GHK-Cu; Glow blend
Plateaued training adaptations	CJC-1295 + Ipamorelin; IGF-1 LR3 (advanced; supervised)

B10. Example Cycles & Stacks (Discuss with Your Provider — No Dosing Listed)

Goal	Structure (Clinic-Neutral Example)
Repair Sprint (6–12 weeks)	BPC-157 + TB500 → transition to BPC-157 maintenance; add KPV if gut/skin inflammation is present; align with PT/strength rehab.
GH-Axis Support (8–12 weeks)	CJC-1295 + Ipamorelin (evening rhythm) ± Super B/omega-3/ADK10 foundation; reassess IGF-1, sleep, body composition.
Mitochondrial Lift (8–12 weeks)	MOTS-C + AICAR cycles; anchor with intervals + strength + protein-forward meals; consider EnerCoQ10/EnerDMG.
Cognitive Clarity Block (4–8 weeks)	Selank daily + NAD+/BDNF/Alpha GPC on work days; Brain Ultra 7 only with close oversight; stop for sleep issues.
Aesthetic Regeneration (8–12 weeks)	Topical/meso GHK-Cu + Glow blend support; pair with protein, collagen, vitamin C, and sun protocol.

B11. Safety, Screening & Monitoring

- Medical oversight: screen for uncontrolled hypertension, active malignancy, pregnancy/breastfeeding, significant psychiatric history, and drug interactions.
- Baseline labs: consider CBC, CMP, fasting glucose/insulin, lipid profile, hs-CRP; specific panels for GH-axis (IGF-1), thyroid, and sex hormones when relevant.
- Side-effect awareness: nausea/flushing (melanocortins), injection site irritation, sleep changes (GH-axis), glucose/lipid shifts; pause and consult if adverse events occur.
- Source quality: insist on COAs (identity, purity), sterility/endotoxin testing, cold-chain or storage as required; avoid unverified online 'research' sources.
- Synergy principle: peptides amplify results when sleep, nutrition, training, and (if indicated) BHRT are aligned; they're not substitutes for fundamentals.

www.ingramcontent.com/pod-product-compliance
Lightning Source LLC
LaVergne TN
LVHW082339200926
848481LV00012B/3390